The Secret Life of Sleep

"Duff leads an absorbing foray into the vibrant activity that we otherwise sleep right through."
Publishers Weekly

"Full of unique insights and surprising facts, this book brings to the fore an entire world that exists behind closed eyes."
Kirkus

"A charmingly written compendium… Duff offers a rich understanding of the subject in which personal insights blend with an amazing array of perspectives in ways that always seem to enhance and complement each other."
Jeannette Mageo – Professor of Anthropology at Washington State University and author of *Dreaming Culture*

THE SECRET LIFE OF SLEEP

KAT DUFF

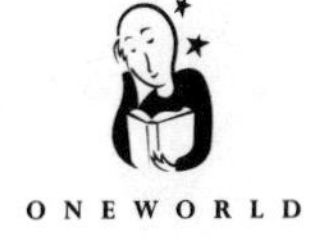

A Oneworld Book

First published in Great Britain and Australia by Oneworld Publications, 2014

Originally published in the United States of America by Beyond Words/Atria Books

A CIP record for this title is available from the British Library

ISBN 978-1-78074-415-5
ISBN 978-1-78074-416-2 (eBook)

Printed and bound by CPI Group (UK) Ltd, Croydon, CRO 4YY

Oneworld Publications
10 Bloomsbury Street
London WC1B 3SR
England

To the worlds within

CONTENTS

One cannot properly describe human life unless
one shows it soaked in the sleep in which it
plunges, which, night after night sweeps round
it as a promontory is encircled by the sea.

—Marcel Proust

Seeing everybody so up all the time made me
think that sleep was becoming pretty obsolete,
so I decided I'd better quickly do
a movie of a person sleeping.

—Andy Warhol

PROLOGUE

Birds do it. Bees do it. Salamanders do it. Even roundworms do it. Giraffes do it standing up. Bats do it hanging upside-down. Sea otters spiral downward like falling leaves. Dolphins do it with one eye open.

To the best of our knowledge, all creatures display some form of sleep behavior, a regular time of quiet when they settle into familiar postures, lose awareness of the outside world, and rest for anywhere from two minutes to twenty hours.[1] The universality of sleep suggests its origins are as old as animal life on earth, an estimated six hundred million years. It also implies that sleep is more than a creature comfort. It is a requirement for life on this planet.

When I was a girl, one night I imagined a world in which we slept only once a year rather than every night. I envisioned hundreds of days pounding out before me like an endless trail of falling dominoes, winding up and over the hills, one day after another without respite. The image filled me with dread—and an enduring appreciation for the gift of sleep.

What did I like so much about sleep? It is hard to distinguish what I feel now from what I felt more than half a century ago, but I remember taking a secret, fiendish delight in the very act of going to bed because I got to shut out the world and say no to everything in it without getting in trouble. It was the only socially sanctioned escape hatch available to me as a child. The sequence of closings that constituted preparing for sleep—putting my clothes away, saying goodnight, shutting the door, turning off the light, covering myself with blankets, closing my eyes—was a ritualized progression toward my own serene departure, each step another stage of letting go and drifting off from the dock, a further phase in my nightly disappearance.

I had a child's love of privacy and invisibility, which sleep undoubtedly satisfied. But there was more. I began to notice that sleep sometimes surreptitiously changed me. When I stayed up late cramming for tests, literally shaking with a growing panic at my inability to remember everything, I inevitably woke up the next morning ready to take the exam. In time, I came to rely upon sleep's uncanny ability to convert my forgetfulness into intelligence, my shakiness into steadiness.

One night, when I was ten or eleven, I dreamed of pinks and greens next to each other, a combination that struck me as unbelievably beautiful, and still does to this day. When I opened my eyes, I continued to see hues rather than objects. My room was no longer a haphazard assortment of books, clothes, and baseball paraphernalia, but an exquisite interplay of colors and shapes playing off of each other like an orchestral piece. Somehow, sleep evoked a capacity for aesthetic appreciation I had never fully experienced before.

There were other times when I awoke from a dream shot through with love or fury toward someone for no apparent reason. At first the feelings seemed ridiculous, and I tried to shrug them off by telling myself it was just a dream. I would often hear that phrase and knew it to mean that something was not real and should be ignored. Sure enough, the feelings usually vanished by the time I stepped onto the school bus. However, there were other times when those seemingly alien emotions stuck with me, and I slowly came to recognize them as true—to me at least. Two of those times are emblazoned into my memory because they signaled enormous changes in my life.

The first happened when I was in secondary school, and I woke from a dream, quivering with rage at my father for reasons unknown to me. I was stunned, confused, and appalled because I admired my father and thought he was the perfect dad. However, in the weeks that followed, I started to notice things I didn't like about him, little things, like the way he dominated the conversation at the dinner table, ignored my brother, and took such pride in his family heritage. Slowly, almost imperceptibly, my idealization of my father faded like a star in a slow-coming dawn.

The second sleep-induced revelation occurred around the same time, when I woke with a feverish sexual desire for a new friend. I had never really considered the possibility of having a sexual life, and the very thought of it, not to mention the experience of it, made my neck and cheeks burn. The urgent press of longing subsided in me as the days passed, but it never went away altogether, even though it was some time before I had the courage to act on it. Whether I liked it or not, my sleep called forth parts of myself I had never known, both clarifying and complicating my life.

When I pondered these experiences, it seemed that my sleeping life was the bigger and more fluid me, and my waking life the smaller, more limited me. One day, paddling out through seaweed into a lake, it occurred to me that our waking selves are like lily pads floating on the surface of our night selves.

It was the insight of an adolescent with time to wonder and

dream. When I grew older and joined the worlds of work and parenting, struggling to find time for everything, I resented wasting precious hours on sleep every night. I viewed my nightly slumber as something like a pit stop in a marathon, a time to pause, recharge, and start again, the way the period at the end of a sentence enables us to stop and take a breath. The sentences were what mattered, not the petty punctuation.

Sleep and waking states are like separate countries with a common border. We cross over twice daily, remembering one world and forgetting the other, inadvertently tracking invisible residues from one into the other. The seemingly unknowable hours we spend in sleep constitute recurring gaps in our waking awareness, and the inescapability of sleep suggests that something important happens during these gaps. It is an occurrence that is so common, so habitual, so ubiquitous, we barely notice. Like the air we breathe, it is something we become aware of only when its quality is deteriorating.

What happens during those missing links between our days? Could these inconspicuous absences shape our lives as surely as the spaces between letters make words readable? My curiosity prompted me to explore that strange phenomenon we call sleep. I began to ask friends, clients, and acquaintances about their sleep, and I quickly found that most people have problems getting the kind or amount they want. Those with physical or psychological problems inevitably slept badly, which makes sense because it is not easy to live with pain, anxiety, or depression in general, not to mention to fall asleep and wake refreshed. What surprised me was the discovery that when the clients I saw as a mental health counselor addressed their sleep problems, their presenting symptoms inevitably became more manageable. Nothing in my training or education as a professional therapist had hinted at that possibility, and it whetted my desire to understand what happens when we lie down and close our eyes.

Sleep is hard to study because it exists, by definition, outside our conscious awareness. Until the middle of the twentieth century, most scientists believed the brain turns off when we fall asleep, only to turn back on upon waking, something like a bedside lamp. Since there was no way to see, feel, or measure the mind asleep, it was easy to assume—and impossible to refute—that nothing happens. Then in 1953, the year DNA was discovered, Eugene Aserinsky placed electrodes on his eight-year-old son while he slept and determined that his brain waves sped up and his eyes darted around under their lids when he was dreaming. That may seem like a simple observation, and Aserinsky later acknowledged that the association between eye movements and dreaming was virtually "common knowledge," but the simultaneous presence of an active brain was new.[2] When Aserinsky and his supervisor, Nathaniel Kleitman, presented their results, it provoked a revolution in scientific thought because it proved that our brains remain active during sleep. Since then, a plethora of new brain-scanning devices have generated a veritable explosion of information elucidating complex and critical processes that occur while we take a break from the outside world. Sleep research has become one of the most diverse and exciting fields of scientific inquiry in the twenty-first century, spawning an abundance of intriguing and conflicting theories.

Of course, dreamers around the world could have told scientists that our minds are active when we sleep; people have been remembering, sharing, and discussing sleep occurrences since the advent of the written word—and no doubt before. It is a different kind of knowledge that has been amassed in the cultural traditions of human life on earth, one that does not necessarily privilege the rationality so valued in the contemporary modernized world but is based on observations made by the multitudes over millennia. People have watched over the sleep of their young children, adult lovers, and dying parents for thousands of years. Hunters, healers, and mystics have cultivated the skills of traveling between realms in sleeplike states to explore and repair their worlds. Even those who do not particularly value their sleep rely upon it for rejuvenation—and occasional revelation.

However, for many people in this day and age, sleep is neither easy nor readily available. When I first told an acquaintance that I was studying sleep, she whipped her head around, fixed her eyes on mine, and growled: "Sleep! What sleep? My sleep is called Ambien!" She is not alone. The National Sleep Foundation (NSF) reports that 25 percent of Americans take some form of sleep medication every night, and that figure does not include evening drinkers.[3] Similarly, in the UK, one in ten people regularly take some form of sleeping pill.[4] Few of us go easily into slumber without something to smooth the way, be it the late show, a nightcap, a bedtime story, or quick sex. And few can wake up the next morning without some form of caffeine, the second most traded commodity on earth next to oil.[5] The "wee small hours of the morning while the whole wide world is fast asleep," as Frank Sinatra crooned in the 1950s, are now lit and roiling with millions of texters, gamers, and midnight emailers. The demands and attractions of our 24/7 global economy are squeezing the hours out of our nights. We are losing the knack—and taste—for rest. Rejuvenating sleep has become as elusive as clean water, dark nights, fresh air, and all the other endangered resources of our natural world.

For many who are desperate for a little more shut-eye, sleep comes with a price tag. A plethora of so-called sleep aids—medications, teas, supplements, eye masks, luxury mattresses, white noise machines, sleep-tracking apps, gentle alarm clocks, and constant positive airway pressure (CPAP) machines promise easy delivery into and out of the hands of sleep. The sleep industry is booming amidst faltering economies worldwide. We would do well to look at what we are losing before it is too late.

Much has been written about the science of sleep in recent years. However, few have ventured far beyond research labs and treatment clinics to tap into the enormous reservoir of human experience on this planet, most of which rarely makes it into academic articles. That body of knowledge expresses itself in the vast array of cultural practices, rituals, oral teachings, proverbs, and lullabies that people around the world have developed over the millennia to fully inhabit the very sleep we rush to leave behind.

In writing this book, I drew upon every source I could lay my hands on: personal experience, scientific research, literary descriptions, autobiographies, myths, sleep and waking routines across cultures and eras, and spiritual traditions from around the globe. Sometimes the observations dovetailed nicely; at other times, they flagrantly contradicted each other. The conflicts have been especially engaging for me because they challenged my assumptions and stretched my powers of comprehension. The topic of sleep opens a Pandora's box of bigger questions about the nature of consciousness and unconsciousness, remembering and forgetting, body and soul, and reality itself, which cannot be ignored.

The chapters that follow are loosely organized to reflect the trajectory of a night's sleep, from the moment we close our eyes to the outside world and descend into the otherworldly realms of slumber and dreams to the moment we rub the sleep from our eyes and return to the waking world. However, each takes a different angle, drawing upon another distinct body of knowledge to reveal the importance of sleep, our need for it, and our so-human efforts to command, control, and even eliminate it from our lives. If there is a theme that threads through these diverse approaches to understanding sleep, it is that our waking and sleeping lives require and inform each other, whether we like it or not. For our waking hours are, as the French novelist Marcel Proust observed, soaked in sleep "as a promontory is encircled by the sea."

I invite you to join me at the shore, where we can peer into the watery depths, tickle our toes in the waves, and leave the dry land of our days behind.

1

WHEN THE SANDMAN COMES: FALLING ASLEEP

A photographer friend of mine once invited me along on an overnight shoot in an old mining town/ski resort in the mountains nearby. It was a chance to get away, see the autumn colors, and spend a night in a historic hotel during the quiet off-season, so I accepted. Unbeknownst to us, however, it was the three-day weekend of Oktoberfest, when Texas universities empty their charges onto the streets of this little town, and for much of the night, young men hold races shouldering full kegs of beer to the whooping and hollering of their friends. The room we were given was right over the Lost Love bar, which had a live band playing that night, and across the street from the Bull O' the Woods Saloon, where the kegs were enjoyed.

There have been times in my life when I could fall asleep anywhere, anytime; but those days are long past, and this particular night gave me ample opportunity to employ all the tricks I have learned over the years to help myself fall asleep. I pulled the curtains shut to block out the street light, plugged in the ear buds of my iPod, stretched out under a warm comforter in the cool air from a cracked window, avoided thinking about aggravating topics—and didn't fall asleep. Finally, I got up, found a crime novel abandoned in a lounge upstairs, and settled down to read the night through. Before long, I had fallen asleep, only to be jolted awake by the sound of my book hitting the floor. When it happened a second time, I decided to try my bed again.

As I padded down the creaky wooden stairs in my socks, it occurred to me that this was the perfect opportunity to observe myself falling asleep and catch as many details of the transition as I could. I slid into bed noting the heaviness in my limbs, my repeated yawning, the tears that slid out the corners of my eyes, my twisting and turning to find the right position under the covers, the flickering of thought-images in that interior space behind my eyelids—and woke up when the band stopped playing at 2:00 AM. I turned over and tried again, this time noticing the sluggishness of my body when I shifted position, my dreamy dimwittedness, a curious, uncaring confusion as to where or who I was... until I was jolted awake by another howl from the street below.

The Sleep Switch

A traditional West African Ashanti tale describes sleep as "The One You Don't See Coming"—the thief you will never be able to catch.[1] Much as we may try, people simply cannot observe themselves in the exact instant of falling asleep. An old German rhyme portrays the effort to catch sleep coming:

> I would like to know how one falls asleep
> Over and over I press myself in the pillow
> And thereby think: "Now I will pay attention."
> But before I have really reflected,

It is already morning,
And I have again awakened.[2]

It is as if a curtain of unconsciousness is swung across the stage, making it impossible to see—or remember—what happens. The ancient Greeks conceptualized this swipe of forgetting as the river of oblivion (Lethe) that circles the cave of sleep (Hypnos) in the underworld. They said that the murmuring waters of Lethe made people drowsy and washed their memories away when they came close to sleep, for in this ancient understanding, sleep required forgetting ourselves in order to enter its inner sanctum.

In 2001, sleep researcher Clifford B. Saper and his colleagues at Harvard University identified a cluster of neurons in the hypothalamus deep inside the brain that triggers sleep onset. This cluster, which they termed a sleep switch, secretes chemicals that effectively shut down wakefulness, including the capacity to be aware of what is happening in the moment, while simultaneously inducing sleep.[3] This switch may be the biological equivalent of the River Lethe.

When we are awake, our brains produce and store a chemical called adenosine triphosphate (ATP) to fuel cell activity. However, as ATP accumulates over the day, it begins to slow down brain activity, making us feel progressively more tired and drowsy. Eventually, with the contribution of other sleep-promoting factors too numerous to mention here, that system-wide state shift we call sleep takes over. As anyone who has pulled an all-nighter can attest, the longer we have been awake previously, the longer and deeper we will sleep to make up for the loss. Scientists propose that a contra-parallel process occurs while we sleep; other chemicals slowly accumulate until we cannot help but wake up and stay awake. It is a homeostatic mechanism that is independent of the cycles of day and night.

Even though we may spend hours approaching sleep, with attending changes in body temperature, brain wave patterns, hormones, and neurotransmitters, the transition from one state to another seems to occur instantly and completely. Noting that sleeping and waking modes appear to be mutually exclusive, Saper and his colleagues theorized that the switch operates likes an on-off, flip-flop toggle, meaning that we are either awake or asleep without much middle ground. The light goes out, as people say, when the switch is flipped, and our brain waves burst into the large oscillations we experience as unconsciousness.

People have often wondered and imagined what flips the switch. In Greek mythology, the god of sleep, Hypnos, taps us with his wand or brushes us with his wings to put us to sleep. In traditional Blackfoot lore, it is a butterfly. In popular European children's stories, the Sandman sprinkles sand or dust on our closed eyes. Whichever way, it takes but a moment, a simple tap, brush, or sprinkle. The experience reminds me of jumping off the high dive—the long climb up the ladder, the tiptoeing back and forth on the board in that familiar push and pull of wanting to jump and being afraid to jump, until the moment seizes us, we leave solid footing, and—a split second later—splash into another world, a wild and watery reality.

Threshold Consciousness

As we wind down and veer toward sleep, we travel through a transitional state called hypnagogia, named after Hypnos. The word literally translates as "sleep driver." There's a parallel transitional state, called hypnopompia, when we wake up. Most of the time, we zip through these states so quickly that we miss them altogether. But occasionally, we pause, as if waiting for the stoplight to turn. During hypnagogia, clusters of neurons take turns shutting down, and sleep creeps over us. Our brain waves slow to a trance-like rhythm, and our attention drifts. When I have engaged in a repetitive task during the day, like playing ping-pong or solitaire, I often see the balls or cards moving into place as soon as I close my eyes. It is called the Tetris effect, after the video game. The effect can also take an audio or kinesthetic form, like feeling the rocking motion of waves after a day of snorkeling.

Hypnagogia and hypnopompia involve more than reliving sensations from daytime activities. People report fleeting visions of geometric patterns; sparks of light or splashes of color; and roaring, hissing, or clanging sounds. Faces may appear with friendly, threatening, or comical expressions. Landscapes unfurl themselves, revealing familiar and otherworldly realms. Sometimes snatches of songs or conversations float by. Virginia Woolf described it well in her novel *To the Lighthouse*:

> As she lost consciousness of outer things… her mind kept throwing up from its depths, scenes, and names, and sayings, and memories, and ideas, like a fountain spurting…

Occasionally, there is the sensation of floating, spinning, or getting bigger or smaller. It is a bizarre reality we slide through between waking and sleeping. The Spanish poet Federico García Lorca once spoke of fairies appearing when mothers sing lullabies to their babies and described seeing one himself once when he was visiting a cousin as a child. Vladimir Nabokov wrote in his autobiography that he would often "become aware of… a neutral, detached anonymous voice which I catch saying words of no importance to me whatever—an English or Russian sentence" just before falling asleep. A friend of mine admitted that she sometimes feels herself swelling up like a balloon until she is as big as the room and then shrinking down to the size of a pea, repeatedly, until she loses all awareness.

Sometimes people startle themselves (and their bedmates) with a massive, involuntary jerk. The scientific name for this phenomenon is myoclonic kick, though it is more commonly known as a sleep start. While it appears to be a primitive reflex generated by the brain stem, no one really knows why we startle like this on the cusp of sleep. Some theorize it is because our brains mistakenly confuse the sudden release of muscle tension, especially among the muscle groups that resist gravity, with a frightening free fall and jerk to stop it, as if grabbing for a branch when tumbling from a tree. Others propose it is left over from the evolutionary need to keep watch for danger, waking us whenever we start to slip off.

Whatever the case, the sensation of dropping suddenly is so strong, people often have split-second dreams of falling, whether it is tripping while running, slipping on ice, tumbling down stairs, or plunging from a precipice. Neurologist Oliver Sacks finds these split-second dreams, which he prefers to call hallucinations, particularly fascinating because they demonstrate how quickly our minds can work to invent a narrative to explain a sensation. In the moment, it seems that the dream has triggered the startle, but it is probably the other way around. Sacks proposes that a "preconscious perception" of the jerk prompts "an elaborate restructuring of time" to provide a story for the event.[4] If he is right, and I suspect he is, our startle dreams are actually cover stories, something like the tales kids spin to explain why the cookies are gone, only more convincing.

These tripping, slipping, tumbling, and plunging dream stories are so common, and so convincing, they have made it into more than a few lullabies. My favorite is the popular "Rock-a-Bye Baby," which has the baby blowing in the wind and falling "cradle and all" at the end. I have always wondered why a lullaby intended to lull an infant to sleep would include such frightening imagery; it seems a cruel thing to give a child heading into the land of Nod. Now I understand. Bedtime is falling time, and these lullabies prepare us for the hallucinations of falling that so often attend the slip into sleep.

Coinciding with the World

For thousands of years, this surreal trance-like state before sleep has been recognized as a place of insight and inspiration. As psychologist Deirdre Barrett documented in her book, *The Committee of Sleep*,[5] nineteenth-century German chemist August Kekulé credited his discovery of the ringed structure of benzene to a hypnagogic vision of circling snakes he had one night while dozing in front of a fire. Eighteenth-century scientist and philosopher Emanuel Swedenborg developed a method for inducing and exploring these states, during which he claimed to have traveled to heaven, hell, and other planets. Salvador Dalí drew inspiration for his paintings from the bizarre imagery of sleep states and recommended eating sea urchins for the best results. Thomas Edison cultivated hypnagogic states to get ideas for new inventions. He would take short naps in the middle of the day while sitting in a chair and holding steel balls in his hands. The moment his muscles relaxed on the brink of sleep, the balls dropped into pie pans, whose clanging woke him instantly—sometimes with a new approach to an old problem.

In 1906, psychoanalyst Herbert Silberer conducted what he called introspective experiments into hypnagogic imagery while falling asleep.[6] To his astonishment, Silberer noted that the images that appeared often related to what he had just been doing. One day, when he tired of trying to improve an awkward passage in an essay he was writing, Silberer closed his eyes and saw himself planing a piece of wood, refining and finishing the shape. On another occasion, after puzzling over something he later admitted was forcing "a problem into a preconceived scheme," he saw himself trying to press a jack-in-the-box back into its box. Over time, Silberer became adept at watching his thoughts transform into a loose array of images and feelings, what Sigmund Freud called primary process thinking. His psychoanalytic orientation gave him a framework for understanding that transformation, making the experience of falling into imagery a familiar, benign, and intriguing one.

However, many are surprised, confused, and even disturbed by the bizarre phenomena that arise at the edge of sleep. The sights, sounds, and sensations can feel so foreign, it is hard to believe they come from inside us, if they do. I have occasionally questioned whether some elements slip in from outside, and the following event made me wonder even more.

I was staying with friends in New Orleans in the midst of a cross-country trip. Dropping off to sleep, I saw a stark black-and-white image of dead cats strewn about an empty street at night. I bolted upright, calmed myself down, and fell back asleep. It happened again, this time with a slightly different view. Every time I went back to sleep that night, there were more dead cats, until I finally got out of bed. Having recently changed my nickname from Kitty to Kat, I thought the visions were telling me that I had died in some way. I poured myself a cup of tea, sat down at the kitchen table, and pondered the implications until dawn. A few hours later, I received a phone call from the friend who was taking care of my cat, FB, while I was away. She told me that she had found FB's body in the street that morning. FB had been run over during the night.

The French philosopher Gaston Bachelard once wrote: "Sleep opens within us an inn for phantoms." While it is not clear whether his phantoms come from within or without the sleeper, he is assured of their fundamental otherness, for he added: "The repose of the night does not belong to us. It is not the possession of our being." The apparition of dead cats that kept intruding upon my sleep that night in New Orleans seems connected—at least in time—to FB's demise in that country lane in western Massachusetts. How that specter found me, and got my attention, is beyond my understanding.

Perhaps there is something about these transitional states that enables us to tune in to dimensions of reality that are ordinarily inaccessible. After all, the hypnagogic state is known to be an impressionable one. Hypnotists regularly induce it in order to circumvent the conscious beliefs of their clients, just as the artists, inventors, and psychologists mentioned above looked to these states to attain insights only available outside their ordinary thinking. Andreas Mavromatis, who published in 1987 what remains the most comprehensive book on hypnagogic experiences, noted that people who share sleeping spaces sometimes report seeing the same images as they drop off, as if the visions were silently passed around in the permeability of near sleep.[7] The French philosopher Jean-Luc Nancy may have explained it best when he described a simultaneity that occurs when falling asleep: "I coincide with the world."[8]

When we lie down, close our eyes, and begin to drift off, we let our guards down and allow ourselves to receive what comes without filtering out the crazy pieces. Our carefully constructed notions of ourselves, of where we end and the world begins, dissolve without our knowing. Startling bits of unknown information may well slip into our minds before the waters of Lethe wash everything away.

2

OPENING THE INN FOR PHANTOMS: SURRENDERING TO SLEEP

One night years ago, when I was living in Austin, Texas, one of my housemates ran into my room, screaming that she had just broken free from something that had landed on her chest as she was falling asleep, smothering her. She had struggled under its weight, unable to breathe, cry out, or move, until it suddenly lifted as quickly as it had landed. I learned later that my friend's experience, called sleep paralysis, is fairly common. While estimates vary considerably, depending on the terminology used and the person asking, people all over the world are familiar with it, and many have had at least one experience with sleep paralysis, calling it many names. The Laotian Hmong people call it dab tsog or *tsog tsuam*, meaning "to crush, press, or smother." A fifty-eight-year-old Hmong gentleman described his experience of dab tsog to researcher Shelley R. Adler in this way: "Suddenly there comes a huge body… It was over me—on my body—and I had to fight my way out of that. I couldn't move—I couldn't talk at all. I couldn't even yell 'No.'"[1]

Charles Dickens, a chronic insomniac, was mystified by the

experience of sleep paralysis, unsure whether to call it waking or sleeping. In *The Adventures of Oliver Twist*, he wrote:

> So far as an overpowering heaviness, a prostration of strength, and an utter inability to control our thoughts or power of motion, can be called sleep, this is it; and yet we have a consciousness of all that is going on about us; and if we dream at such a time, words which are really spoken, or sounds which really exist at the moment, accommodate themselves with surprising readiness to our visions, until reality and imagination become so strangely blended that it is afterwards almost a matter of impossibility to separate the two.

In his famous story *A Christmas Carol*, Dickens portrayed Scrooge's encounters with the ghost of Marley as the telltale features of a hypnopompic visitation: the sense of a presence in the room, the ominous sounds of footsteps and chains clanking, and the dreamer's clear awareness of being awake in a particular space and time. Given how common and universal experiences of sleep paralysis are, it is a wonder the phenomenon has not attracted more attention or study. Medical anthropologist David J. Hufford, who has been researching the subject for decades, notes that experiences of sleep paralysis were well-known and discussed in the West until the advent of the Enlightenment in the seventeenth century. During the past three hundred years, he explains, knowledge of the experience was "erased... from the cultural repertoire," as it came to be considered a sign of primitive ignorance or madness.[2] As a result, many living in the West have been afraid to admit, much less to discuss, having the experience for fear of being labeled.

The Spirit Sent to Suffocate Sleepers

Throughout history and across the globe, people have reported encounters with beings that watch, threaten, or attack when the sleeper is awake but unable to move.[3] They have been called angels, demons, incubi, werewolves, hags, ghosts, fairies, djinns, aliens, and more. The word *nightmare* itself is derived from *mara*, a Scandinavian term that refers to "a spirit sent to torment or suffocate sleepers," also known as the crusher. Most hypnagogic visitations are terrifying, variously described as ghost oppression, witch riding, demon possession, or alien encounters.

While these experiences appear to have a biological basis, they are difficult to study because they occur in virtually every culture (some of which discourage their discussion), are described in the words of innumerable native languages, and cannot be made to appear upon command in a sleep lab. Our scientific understanding of sleep, which is based primarily on research conducted among middle-class Westerners in laboratory studies, cannot adequately encompass the cultural diversity of sleep patterns, including those of sleep paralysis experiences.

Despite this limitation, most researchers agree with the scientific speculation that sleep paralysis occurs when the mechanisms of dream sleep have paralyzed our voluntary muscles while we are awake, usually when falling asleep or waking up. It is often considered to be a dream intrusion into waking life, occurring most often at the threshold between the two. This explanation accounts for the complex cluster of sensations commonly described: the inability to move or speak, the difficulty breathing, and the fantastic imagery. The cluster "fits well with a narrative of assault by a strange intruder," as prominent sleep paralysis researcher J. Allan Cheyne and his associates at the University of Waterloo in Ontario noted in 1999.[4] However, Hufford suggests that the cross-cultural consistency and reliable replicability of the sense of a terrifying spirit presence during sleep paralysis imply there is more to it than biology can explain at this point.[5]

It could be that our brains unconsciously concoct a story to explain the physiological sense of alarm in finding oneself awake and paralyzed with just the shallow breathing of light sleep. Our minds are always theorizing about what is happening, trying to explain things to us. One night, when I woke up to the sound of soft, padding footsteps downstairs, my mind launched into a variety of possible explanations: my partner is going to the bathroom, a thief is looking for silver, or a raccoon got in through the cat door. That is what brains do. They invent plausible stories from the limited information we have. When neurologist Patrick McNamara wondered what the source of the "sensed presence" might be, he posed the possibility that our brains may have an "automatic predator-detector" circuit that creates the sense of a malevolent presence when triggered to ensure our rapid response.[6] A mechanism like this would have a clear evolutionary advantage, even if it gets misapplied at times.

In 2006, neuropsychiatrist Shahar Arzy and his colleagues at the University of Geneva applied focused electrical stimulation on the left side of the head of an epileptic patient in hopes of reducing her seizures.[7] To everyone's surprise, she immediately felt the presence of "an illusory shadow person" in the room. The section of her brain that was stimulated handles the processing of information about one's position in space, and whenever she moved, the shadow person made the same movement. The study has been cited as evidence that out-of-body experiences and hypnagogic visitations are actually self-images dislocated in space, illusions created by our brains under stress. Regardless of what causes these frightening experiences, they are real to those who behold them. Most cultures provide practices—prayers, amulets, locks, or communal sleeping arrangements—to ward off visitations in the borderland between waking and sleeping, for the nearness of sleep dismantles our daytime defenses, and renders us naked and vulnerable.[8]

The Nightly Annihilation

When we prepare for sleep, we strip ourselves of the accoutrements of selfhood: our clothes, glasses, makeup, and false teeth. We bid goodbye to the people around us, lie down in stillness, and return to our original, solitary nakedness. As Heraclitus, the ancient Greek philosopher, observed: "The waking have one common world, but the sleeping turn aside each into a world of his own." Once the lights are off, and our eyes closed, even the world, as we've known it, vanishes, and the familiar "I" evaporates. It is the nightly annihilation of daytime awareness, what Shakespeare called "the death of each day's life." Some find this daily wrenching from the waking world to be an intolerable "betrayal of reason, humanity, genius," to quote author Vladimir Nabokov. Thomas Edison called it "an absurdity, a bad habit." For brilliant minds and prodigious achievers like Nabokov and Edison, succumbing to sleep can feel like defeat. After all, it requires that we put down our tools, relinquish our ambitions, and submit to something we cannot control or even put off for another day. Others yearn for the erasure of slumber—for them, the murmuring waters of forgetting are salve to sore hearts and tired bodies. None are more eloquent about this longing than the insomniac. "O bed! O bed! Delicious bed!" wrote the English poet Thomas Hood, "That heaven on earth to the weary head."

Whether we welcome or resist sleep, there is no escaping it. The longer we go without sleep, the stronger its power to overcome us, even when we are doing something else. Brief episodes of what sleep scientists call microsleep, which last anywhere from a fraction of a second to thirty seconds, begin to intrude upon our waking awareness, forcing heads to nod and eyelids to droop, often without our knowing it.[9] This is why it is so dangerous to drive or operate machinery when we are sleepy; unbeknownst to us, secret snatches of sleep impair our ability to remain vigilant and respond quickly. We are understandably most prone to these intrusions at night because sunset prompts the secretion of the sedative hormone melatonin, compromising our capacity for alertness. Even chronic insomniacs, who insist they have lain awake all night, drop into sleep for invisible spans of time, as lab studies reveal. It is impossible to walk the fine tightrope of waking awareness without slipping—repeatedly—into the slumbering sea below.

There is an affinity between falling asleep and dying that cannot be ignored. In fact, the word *sleep* is commonly used as a euphemism for "death"; we speak of putting a pet to sleep, rather than admitting we have asked a veterinarian to (kindly) kill him or her. As the Spanish writer Cervantes noted: "There is very little difference between a man in his first sleep, and a man in his last sleep." Both involve lying down and staying still. In so doing, we give up verticality, the tension between up and down, inside and outside, the oppositions that characterize being awake. Conscious awareness, our constant companion by day, abandons us.

Sleep and death have long been linked. In the ancient Greek cosmology, Hypnos, the god of Sleep, and Thanatos, the god of Death, are twin brothers. Across the Mediterranean in Egypt, sleep was considered to be a daily rehearsal for death because a person's unique spiritual aspect, portrayed as a falcon with a human head, was thought to separate from the body in sleep as it does in death. The Talmud describes sleep as one-sixtieth part of death, the fraction understood to be the threshold of perception for Jewish legal purposes.[10] In other words, sleep proffers the faintest perceptible glimpse of death available to the living. In some Hindu and Buddhist traditions, sleep is viewed as a spiritual practice that prepares us for the shifts in consciousness required after death, teaching us to withdraw first from the outer world of objects, then the inner world of thoughts and images, until we reach the blissful nothingness of deep, dreamless sleep.[11] The Tibetan physician Yeshi Dhonden put it simply: "In the Buddhist view, sleep and death states are similar."[12]

It comes as no surprise then, that bedtime prayers inevitably address the mortal dangers of sleep, like the popular one that follows, first recorded in 1160 AD:

Now I lay me down to sleep
I pray the Lord my soul to keep
If I should die before I wake
I pray the Lord my soul to take.

I am partial to a traditional Scottish bedtime prayer I wish I had known when my stepdaughter was young and afraid to go to sleep:

From ghoulies and ghosties
And long-legged beasties
And things that go bump in the night
Good Lord, Deliver us![13]

Lullabies, like the following verse from Brahms, often reassure sleepers that they are protected when disappearing behind closed eyes:

Sleepyhead, close your eyes,
Mother's right here beside you,
I'll protect you from harm,
You'll awake in my arms.
Guardian angels are near,
So sleep on, with no fear.
Guardian angels are near,
So sleep on, with no fear.

Sleep Dread

When I was in third grade, my elderly grandfather died at home in a hospital bed while my brother and I were playing upstairs in the attic before Sunday dinner. Since my father had just told us to quiet down because Grandpa Burt was sleeping in the room below, I concluded that I had killed him. I also decided that the police would come to arrest me when I was sleeping and take me away to jail for the rest of my life. So I packed my little suitcase, placed it next to my bed, and waited for their arrival, night after night, all the while crying over the ruin I had made of my life. Fortunately, when the police never came, I figured they had forgotten about me and put my suitcase back in the wardrobe.

What I find so curious about this memory is the fact that my dread and guilt abandoned me by day, only to grab hold of me when it was time for bed. The social milieu of family and school life carried me along while the sun was up—even when my teacher became convinced that my red, puffy eyes were a sign of the chicken pox and sent me home, even when my mother drove me right back to school insisting I wasn't sick. I was fine through it all. I did not think about spending the rest of my life in prison, and it never occurred to me to tell either of them that the police were coming for me. But at night, when I closed the door to my room, turned off the light, and approached my bed, I felt a terrible sickening as my thoughts returned and fixated on the details of my demise. Perhaps it was the darkness itself that robbed me of my daytime assurances and securities. Or the aloneness. There was something about being by myself in the night, having to push away from the familiar day world in order to fall asleep, that sent me to my knees before God.

Fear of falling asleep has two technical names in the parlance of sleep disorders: hypnophobia and somniphobia. Children are most vulnerable to this, famously afraid of all manner of monsters that could be lurking in the darkness of their bedrooms. The terror of being left alone beyond the safety of light is a primitive one with a clear evolutionary advantage; young ones left to fend for themselves were easy prey and most likely did not survive to pass on their genes. However, children do not usually display these terrors until two or three years old, although they often struggle with them for years to come, despite the plethora of kids' books intended to allay nighttime anxieties. Child development experts like to comfort parents by explaining that bedtime resistance is a common, normal phase youngsters undergo, a function of vivid imaginations coupled with difficulties distinguishing fantasy from reality.

However, there may be more to it. Ira Glass, the host of the popular radio program *This American Life*, reported that he began fearing sleep when he was six years old and his uncle was drafted to Vietnam.[14] Glass lay awake nights worrying that his uncle would die and that he would surely be drafted and killed when he came of age as well. There are a myriad of frightening sights, scary stories, awful silences, and baffling explanations that kids grapple with daily, not to mention the fundamental tasks of coming to terms with their vulnerability and the fact of death. While we would like to dismiss their fears as childish, it is important to remember that children are dealing with profound existential questions, challenges that do not disappear when they grow up. We all experience some trepidation in the face of life's uncertainties, and research on fatigue and stress indicates that our capacity to manage our distress diminishes the later it gets and the more tired we are.[15] The only advantage adults have over children when it comes to facing these challenges is experience and (hopefully) a few more coping skills.

A surprising number of adults struggle against sleep. Some have had traumatic experiences while sleeping—a house fire, for example, a break-in, or an assault—and remain hypervigilant thereafter. Others are plagued by hypnagogic visitations, nightmares, hazardous episodes of sleepwalking, or fear of bed bugs. Still others worry they will stop breathing, lose control of their bladders, or not be able to sleep or wake up, and they approach their beds with the sense of impending doom. An acquaintance once told me that as a child, she often felt herself to be stretched out on a sled at the top of a snowy mountain when she lay down and closed her eyes, and she dreaded the moment, which always seemed to come, when she would start sliding, faster and faster, charging into a thickly wooded area where she was sure to crash into a tree and die, alone. The expectation would keep her awake for hours as a child, and it instilled a terror of falling asleep that has never left her.

No one is looking out for us in sleep. We are existentially alone and required to give ourselves over to something we cannot know or even recall the next day. It takes an act of faith to fall asleep, and not everyone has it. A friend of mine repeatedly wakes herself up the moment she has an irrational thought at the edge of sleep, despite her desperate need and wish for rest. Her nights are epic battles between her intentional efforts to calm, relax, and ready for sleep and her instinctual ever-vigilant reflexes that will not let her drop off. Even when we manage to sleep, fear can circle our beds. An adolescent friend told me once that when her dog curls up at the end of her bed, she sleeps soundly because she knows her dog will protect her, but when her dog is gone and her baby brother sleeps with her, she wakes up every time he moves to make sure he is okay.

Many people living in tribal societies consider sleep to be a dangerous time during which our spirits can depart our bodies, leaving us vulnerable to physical and spiritual predation.[16] This is why people rarely, if ever, sleep alone in tribal cultures, and many regard the contemporary Western practice of having children sleep by themselves tantamount to criminal neglect.[17] Even if they manage to evade the clutches of bears and witches while their eyes are closed, their wandering spirits may not make it back into their bodies before morning. I have often had the experience of waking up feeling disoriented, frightened, or sick, feeling as though I have lost some part of myself, and I scramble to collect myself. The very phrase *collect myself* implies we are capable of scattering and losing pieces of ourselves. Just as it takes faith to fall asleep, we may also need the grace of the gods to make it through sleep intact and unharmed. Waking up alive and whole is a special dispensation not to be taken for granted, which in part explains the common practice of morning prayers. A traditional Jewish morning prayer (*Modeh ani l'fanecha melech chai v'kayam sh'hechezarta bi nishmati b'chemla rabah emunatecha*) translated into English reads:

I am thankful before You,
Living and Sustaining Ruler,
Who returned my soul to me with mercy.
Your faithfulness is great.[18]

Safe Sleep

Throughout history, people have gone to enormous lengths to ensure the safety of their sleep. In traditional hunter-gatherer societies, family members nestle together; keep fires to shed light, provide warmth, and smoke out the insects; wake frequently to check for danger; and tell stories or play music. Safety derives from being literally embedded with familial others, even domesticated animals.[19] In many modern Northern European and American households, people retreat to separate residences, lock doors, retire to rooms designed for sleeping alone or in conjugal pairs, turn out lights, and cover themselves with layers of bedding. Here, safety comes from a dark, quiet, guarded solitude.

In the West, people have developed elaborate bedtime rituals, especially for children. There are after-dinner baths, followed by changing into special night apparel, reading stories, singing lullabies, cuddling stuffed animals, giving goodnight kisses, and turning on night lights—all to provide a sense of security. Even adults have comforting, customary ways of readying themselves for sleep, be it watching the ten o'clock news, checking email, or reading in bed. One of my favorite childhood memories is of listening to my mother play solitaire on the dining room table late at night. The slapping, sliding, and swooshing of cards brought both of us to the threshold of sleep. Even my brother clearing his asthmatic throat became soothing by virtue of its regularity.

While sleep is often viewed as a strictly biological event, cultures clearly play an important role in defining and providing the sense of safety it requires. Individuals, families, and communities, even those that have spread far and wide, have unique cultural practices to prepare for sleep. My Hispanic friend sleeps with her baby in the living room while her husband shares a bed with their toddler to ensure that all the little ones are carefully attended. My middle-aged neighbor keeps his computer and television on all night to follow foreign stock markets and sleeps fitfully on the living room sofa to keep from waking his wife in the bedroom. Down the street, a young social worker and her husband share a mattress on the floor with their babies while their dogs protect the household.

If I asked any of them why they sleep in the manner they do, they would probably answer that it only makes sense, but their sleep solutions only make sense according to their values and the cultural contexts in which they live. As these examples suggest, nowhere is the influence of culture more evident in the experience of sleep than in the care parents give to the sleep of their young children.

3

CRIBS, CRADLES, AND SLINGS: SLEEPING BABIES ACROSS CULTURES

I have always had a certain fondness for the rituals that go with putting a child to bed, especially the moments of sleepy intimacy they foster, so I was surprised to learn that the notion of a bedtime is not the norm around the world, even among other industrialized societies. For example, in Southern European countries like Italy, Spain, and Greece, children are typically allowed to participate in the family's late evening life, falling asleep in cars or laps instead of their own rooms, and there is no specified time for going to bed. The same is often true for families in Central and South America. In many tribal cultures, such as the Maya or the Balinese, infants and toddlers are held, carried, or accompanied continuously by a series of caretakers. They are able to doze, fall asleep, stir, and waken under many circumstances, even in the middle of noisy, all-night ritual observances, with little need for special sleep aids like dummies, blankets, or stuffed animals.[1]

In their seminal 2002 review of cross-cultural sleep practices, anthropologists Carol Worthman and Melissa Melby found that, in general, sleepers in Westernized, postindustrial countries have routine times for bed and waking to accommodate work or school, while traditional, non-Westernized sleepers have more fluid sleep schedules, moving in and out of sleep in the course of a day.[2] They also discovered that in most cultures around the world (in Asia, Africa, Central and South America, Southern Europe, and parts of Scandinavia), children sleep within arm's reach of other family members, what anthropologists term co-sleeping, despite colonial efforts to encourage indigenous peoples to develop solitary sleep arrangements. They do not necessarily sleep in the same bed, but they are near enough to each other to observe movements and hear sounds, even muffled ones. Only in the societies of Northern mainland Europe and America, and to some extent the places colonized by those powers, has sleep been both reliably compressed into a single stretch of time and become a private affair necessitating bedtime rituals.

A History of Consolidated, Solitary Sleep

The contemporary Western pattern of sleep, characterized by one long, uninterrupted bout of sleep a day in a quiet, darkened room apart from others (with 62 percent reporting difficulty sleeping a few nights a week)[3] is a fairly recent invention—and unique to some industrialized nations. Historian A. Roger Ekirch made the remarkable discovery that up until the Industrial Age, most Europeans experienced two spans of sleep per night, with an hour or two of quiet wakefulness between.[4] It is unlikely that anyone, adult or child, expected to sleep through the night. This middle-of-the-night waking time, called the watch or vigil, provided the opportunity to smoke a pipe, ponder a dream, brew a tub of ale, make love, or visit. It was highly valued in Medieval Europe as a time of calm relaxation, when thoughts and perceptions mingled with dreams.

Nighttime itself was understood to be a separate season, an alternate reign, that defied conventional daytime values. It was not a passive, empty state but one of a different kind of activity—a state of socializing, scheming, and fooling around in the freedom darkness affords. The pattern of divided or segmented sleep began to disappear in cities during the late 1700s and virtually vanished under the onslaught of industrialization, which required long hours of work outside the home. To accommodate these demands in accordance with standardized clock time, sleep was compressed, or consolidated, into one stretch per night. It was not an easy transition; employers used rewards, threats, and fines to make their workers get to work on time and toil until the bell rang at the end of the day. To this day, many indigenous peoples struggle against the imposition of clock time.[5]

Communal sleep was also the standard before the modern era, especially among middle and lower classes. Peasant families even brought their farm animals under their roofs, still a practice in many traditional societies. Besides providing protection from intruders, animals generated additional warmth. Babies slept with adults, and virtually everyone shared a bed with someone else.[6] The use of phrases like *bedfellows* and *night companions* in medieval texts suggests that bed sharing was a popular practice, one that cultivated both intimacy and equality between householders. Middle-class homes rarely designated separate rooms for sleeping or eating; almost any room could be used for conducting private or public affairs.

Travelers, even if they were strangers, often shared a bed. A Virginia tavern dating back to the Colonial era had a sign posted next to the beds reading: "No more than six can sleep in a bed."[7] Communal sleeping was a necessity for those with one-room homes and limited bedding but also a preference for many, one that continued well into the twentieth century. In fact, a series of studies conducted between 1989 and 1996 indicated that contemporary Hispanic, African American, and immigrant peoples living in Western countries are much more likely to co-sleep with their infants than Caucasians are.[8]

French historian Jean-Louis Flandrin pointed out that the communal bed was the only gathering place for families, apart from the table, for centuries; as such, it was an important source of domestic cohesion, as it still is among many indigenous cultures, especially on ceremonial occasions. The Maori in New Zealand retain collective sleeping as a form of cultural resistance, citing their proverb: "Eat with us and sleep with us; then you will know our lifestyle."[9] In the modern world, young people seem to be carrying on the tradition, lounging around on their beds and visiting with friends. What parent has not come home to find a heap of tangled bodies on their child's bed, reportedly studying?

From Cradles to Cribs

Infants and young children continued to sleep with their mothers in the West throughout the 1700s, either in the parental bed or next to it in a cradle. When infants outgrew the cradle, they typically moved into a trundle bed pulled out from under the parents' bed. When houses got bigger in the 1700s, freestanding cribs began to replace the trundle bed. Babies were also carried by their caregivers in arms or slings, even during work, until the Industrial Age. When Queen Victoria purchased three push-style baby carriages in the 1840s, she started a fad among the upper classes that has never gone away.[10] American and British babies now spend two-thirds of their time physically separate from their caretakers, in strollers, car seats, high chairs, cribs, and swings.

In the 1890s, Americans were encouraged by professionals to stop putting their babies in cradles next to the parental bed and start using stationary cribs that could be placed in a separate room. The rationale given was that solitary sleep would reduce stimulation and cultivate the child's independence. Attachment between mother and child was seen as a sign of weakness—an attitude that continued in professional circles throughout the nineteenth century and much of the twentieth in Northern European and American cultures most influenced by Anglo-Saxon traditions. Experts also feared for the safety of infants in the family bed, given rumors that some mothers rolled on top of their babies and suffocated them to limit family size. The child's nursery, which started as a nook adjoining the parent's bedroom, became a separate bedroom for the child. It was a sign of prosperity to be able to afford another room, a convenience for parents, and privacy for all. It also marked a break with the ancient, species-wide tradition of maintaining twenty-four-hour contact between mother and infant for at least the first year of life.

Sleep began to be viewed as something children need to learn how to do; it was no longer understood to be a natural self-regulating, biological process. Experts wrote baby care manuals prescribing strict sleep and feeding schedules and warned caregivers not to kiss or cuddle babies for fear of transmitting disease. Once most of the diseases that had previously taken the lives of many newborns were under control, medical professionals proffered the same advice, but now it was for the infant's psychological well-being. They counseled parents not to give in to their baby's cries for comfort or feeding for fear of spoiling them.

Well into the twentieth century, the United States Children's Bureau claimed that "a baby is never to inconvenience the adult," and giving in to an infant's cries upon separation "would make a spoiled, fussy baby, and a household tyrant."[11] The advice was based on the importance of independence, the prioritization of the parental relationship, and the need to avoid the appearance of improper sexual relations. Some parents went so far as to sedate their babies with opiates to keep them from crying at night, until the practice was outlawed in the 1920s.

In the first half of the twentieth century, when artificial light became available in cities and police arrived to patrol the streets at night, parents began to enjoy evening activities apart from their children, further establishing the practice of an early bedtime and solitary sleep for their little ones. After World War II, the progressive pediatrician Dr. Spock encouraged parents to be more flexible, affectionate, and playful with their children but still recommended minimal contact between mother and baby during the night.[12] Breast-feeding was rapidly declining at the time, and in the mid-1950s, seven Midwestern women responded by founding La Leche League to provide mother-to-mother education and support for breast-feeding, asserting that the baby's need for ongoing physical contact is as strong as his or her need for food. In spite of their efforts, separate sleep became the norm for children in the United States and the UK.

Before long, an infant's ability to sleep alone until morning became a developmental milestone expected of all, despite the fact that many poor or immigrant families secretly continued to practice shared sleeping arrangements by necessity and/or cultural tradition. In the middle of the twentieth century, English pediatrician Donald Winnicott observed that children frequently used special transitional objects, like blankets, stuffed animals, or dummies, to comfort themselves in the absence of a parent, especially when falling asleep or waking in the night. These cherished possessions, which served to replace the mother's body, became so ubiquitous in Western industrialized cultures that child psychologists started to identify their use as emblematic of a natural stage through which all children pass.

Anthropologists have begun to challenge their assumptions, pointing out that children raised in cultures where parents and infants sleep within arm's reach have much less use for transitional objects. For example, in Korea, where co-sleeping is an established tradition, fewer than one in five babies cling to a cherished belonging to fall asleep, while the vast majority of American infants clutch teddy bears and the like in their cribs.[13] A 2006 review of cross-cultural literature concluded that infants tend to use sleep aids when they are expected to fall asleep on their own, regardless of culture.[14] A child's dependence on transitional objects may be more of a demonstration of his or her creative resourcefulness in satisfying needs for physical contact than an innate behavior or developmental stage. Unlike transitional objects, however, the one sleep aid that has been used for thousands of years across the globe and continues to be popular among both parents and children is the lullaby.

Easing into Sleep

Four thousand years ago, in what is now Iraq, someone scratched the words of a lullaby, "Little Baby in the Dark House," into a clay tablet small enough to fit in the palm of your hand.[15] While the melody is unknown, the song shares many of the features of lullabies found around the world today: simple wording, repeating phrases, and a rhythm that mimics a swinging or rocking motion.

Some lullabies dispense with words altogether, like the popular Irish lullaby, "Too-Ra-Loo-Ra-Loo-Ral," allowing the hardworking language centers of a child's brain to let go as it relies on the sounds to soothe. Others make promises or offer bribes: sweet dreams, the protection of angels, mockingbirds, and more if only the child will just fall asleep. Still others tell stories and engage the child in flights of imagination, cultivating that dreamy, floating quality of near sleep. "Wynken, Blynken, and Nod," one of my favorites, is a great example:

> Wynken, Blynken, and Nod one night
> Sailed off in a wooden shoe…
> All night long their nets they threw
> To the stars in the twinkling foam—
> Then down from the skies came the wooden shoe,
> Bringing the fishermen home…
> And some folk thought 'twas a dream they'd dreamed
> Of sailing that beautiful sea—
> But I shall name you the fishermen three:
> Wynken,
> Blynken,
> And Nod.
>
> Wynken and Blynken are two little eyes,
> And Nod is a little head,
> And the wooden shoe that sailed the skies
> Is a wee one's trundle-bed.
> So shut your eyes while Mother sings
> Of wonderful sights that be,
> And you shall see the beautiful things
> As you rock in the misty sea,
> Where the old shoe rocked the fishermen three:
> Wynken,
> Blynken,
> And Nod.[16]

Lullabies like these may be the prototypes for contemporary

guided visualizations and progressive relaxations that gently lead the listener down the path toward sleep with a soft, lulling voice. Older, more traditional lullabies are often not so pleasant, however. Many do not protect the child from the ways of the world at all; instead, they plunge him or her into the thick of it, warning of wolves, hyenas, or drunken men, recounting terrible tragedies or a mother's miseries, not unlike the fearsome mysteries many contemporary adults read before bed. Perhaps they work by acknowledging our fears, containing them in a familiar format and the voice of the mother or writer. Maybe they function to instruct and prepare us for life's challenges. Then again, they may simply soothe by fostering an emotional communion, an empathetic connection, between the singer and the listener.

An old Gaelic lullaby from southern Denmark, *Mues sang fa Hansemand* ("Mother's Song to Little Hans"), depicts the grim realities of their family life. It starts by telling little Hans: "Be quiet now, my little boy / Please lie down to sleep," adding "Mum is so very tired / She badly needs to rest." The lullaby proceeds to explain that Dad and Mum have to work very hard to earn a living, and the children suffer as a result. The lullaby continues: "Hans cries again and again" when Mum has to leave. Mum and Dad wish they could give Hans better, but they cannot. [17]

The grief, guilt, and rage found in this song often surface in lullabies, especially those sung by oppressed and depressed caregivers, including the nannies, au pairs, and slaves saddled with caring for other people's babies at the expense of their own. Lullabies can be as much for the mother as for the child, offering an extraordinarily intimate communication that is often barred from daytime interactions. Since babies take their cues from their caregivers, anything that can help a sad and tired mother unburden herself would, most likely, also calm the little one listening. Even though the words of this lullaby evoke grievous sorrow, I imagine that the aching rhythm and its tender tones override the story to smooth anxious brows, which may be what we all need when it is time for sleep. It is not easy to let go and drop into sleep, and we often need facilitators, what the sleep industry likes to call sleep aids, to help us along. The presence of a trusted companion, and the contact of touch, small talk, or goodnight wishes, is one of the best.

Whether it is an old shoe rocking on ocean waves or a cradle swinging from a tree, the steady rhythm of swaying also seems to help lull people to sleep. The motion is reminiscent of what it feels like to be carried inside the belly of an expectant mother or on the hip of a new one. In 2001, neuroscientists at the University of Geneva rigged up a bed so it would sway gently and then invited a dozen research subjects to nap on it while scalp electrodes recorded their brain activity.[18] As predicted, they found that people fell asleep faster when the bed was rocking. They also discovered, much to their surprise, that subjects slept more deeply and felt more refreshed upon waking. Noting that deep sleep fosters memory formation and brain plasticity, they wondered if rocking beds could help recovery from strokes or head injuries. As of 2011, the team of neuroscientists was planning to continue research in this area.

Of course, people have been finding and creating ways to rock to sleep for ages. More than a thousand years ago, the Mayans of Central America invented woven sleeping nets, or hammocks, which quickly spread along trade routes in the Americas, including the Caribbean islands. Christopher Columbus was so taken with them, he brought several back to Spain in the late 1400s.[19] In Europe, fathers hollowed out logs to make the first baby cradles, which could be hung from trees to swing in the wind or jiggled with a foot on the floor. To this day, the vast majority of infants in Thailand begin their sleep journeys in swinging or rocking cradles.[20]

I once house-sat for a friend in New Orleans whose bed (a mattress on a four-by-eight sheet of plywood) swung from the ceiling suspended by ropes attached to the four corners. It was hard to get into because the bed would not stay still, but once I learned how to leap onto the mattress, falling asleep while gently swinging felt absolutely delicious. Every time I turned over, the bed started swaying again. It felt like being in a boat rocked by waves.

Classical Chinese contained several words and phrases for falling asleep, including *jui zhen*, "to approach the cushion," *qin* and *wo*, "to lie down," *jiao jie*, "to join the eyelashes," and *an*, *xi*, and *xiu*, "to rest," each identifying a step in the process.[21] In going through the motions, completing each step, we follow an ancient, instinctual rhythm, though clothed in the particulars of a given culture. It reminds me of the movements my dog makes as she prepares herself a bed in the dirt; scratching vigorously at first, circling round and round, gradually slowing until, like a top, she finally drops.

Lullabies and rocking rhythms may work well to lull a baby to sleep, but they do not always keep that child asleep. As many a parent will tell you, the moment you lie back down and fall asleep, the baby inevitably starts to scream.

Crying to Sleep

When I was in elementary school, my grandmother began inviting a friend of hers who had a granddaughter my age for tea on the first Sunday of every month. We granddaughters were assigned to play together for the afternoon while they had tea and talked. My once-a-month friend always wanted to play a game she called Mommy Baby. It went like this: I was Baby, and she was Mommy.

Mommy puts Baby to bed, kisses her goodnight, and leaves the room. Baby cries, "Waaa! Waaa!" and Mommy storms back in, smacks Baby upside the head, and shouts: "Be quiet!"

Putting baby to sleep is a common feature of children's play, but I didn't like her version and repeatedly tried to convince my friend to switch roles or play another game, to no avail. She insisted on re-enacting her script every time we saw each other. Once the scenario was ritually enacted, we were free to play as other children do. This went on for years. Why it never occurred to me to tell an adult, I'll never know. It was one of those secrets-till-we-die things that children do.

Nighttime crying is hardly a new phenomenon, and it is undoubtedly one of the most trying aspects of parenting young children. The ancient Babylonian lullaby, "Little Baby in the Dark House" addressed the issue from the very start: "You have seen the sun rise. Why are you crying? Why are you screaming?"[22] It continues by telling the child that he or she has disturbed the house god, who then shouts: "Who has disturbed me?... Who has scared me?" The lullaby answers: "The baby has disturbed you. The baby has scared you, making noises like a drunkard who cannot sit still on his stool." The lullaby ends with the house god commanding: "Call the baby now!"

The issue of how to handle a baby's night cries is hotly debated by contemporary parents, pediatricians, and child development experts in the United States, Canada, Germany, the United Kingdom, and other countries with Germanic and Anglo-Saxon traditions. On one side is the popular Ferber method (also known as graduated extinction), which advocates putting babies six months or older to sleep at standard times with comforting routines and leaving them there for increasingly longer periods until they manage to sleep on their own.[23] The idea is that babies learn to self-soothe, to tolerate and reduce the distress of finding themselves alone in the dark when they are not repeatedly fed or rocked back to sleep. When they cry, parents are advised to wait before entering the room, and offer verbal reassurance only, before leaving. Ferber advocates claim that a few nights of this procedure usually prompts babies to sleep until morning. It is an approach that is welcomed by many working and sleep-deprived parents desperate for a full night of sleep. At the extreme, without the comforting routines and graduated steps recommended by Dr. Ferber, it is called the cry-it-out method.

On the other side, attachment-oriented (or evolutionary) parenting experts counter that these methods silence babies and accustom them to abandonment.[24] They point out that ever since humans evolved as hunter-gatherers some three million years ago, newborns have lived on, or next to, the bodies of their mothers who nursed them when needed, a practice that continues in many nonindustrialized communities to this day. At night, infants snuggled up with parents and siblings who quickly responded to their cries so as not to attract predators. Evolutionary biologists theorize that when humans became upright long ago, the time babies spent in utero was shortened to accommodate the narrowed pelvises required for walking. As a result, human newborns continued gestation after birth, and mother-infant skin-to-skin-contact became their natural habitat.[25] Even though babies are now safe from most predators, their physiology may still expect conditions that were the norm for thousands of years when life was a battle for survival.

Jean Liedloff, an American writer who spent two and a half years living deep in the Venezuelan jungle with a contemporary hunter-gatherer tribe, the Yequana Indians, carefully observed infant sleep, noting:

> [The infant] is asleep most of the time, but even as he sleeps,

> he is becoming accustomed to the voices of his people, to the sounds of their activities, to the bumpings, jostlings, and moves without warning… and the safe, right feel of being held to a living body… He is feeling right, therefore he rarely has any need to signal by crying.[26]

When Liedloff remarks that the infant "rarely has any need to signal by crying," she is referring to the fact that all mammals, including humans, cry when they are separated from their caretakers for any length of time. These cries, known as "distress vocalizations," can usually be distinguished from other ones by their vehemence because they display a physiological state of alarm, the activation of what neuroscientist Jaap Panksepp calls the panic system.[27] Panksepp theorizes that the panic system evolved from older pain mechanisms to ensure that adults care for their infants.

One of the trickiest things about the contemporary expectation that children sleep through the night is that it involves a lengthy separation—some would say an abandonment—which triggers alarm for both parent and child. A baby's cries are so painful to hear, most caretakers cannot help but respond by soothing the child. Comforting responses release opioids in the bodies of both parties, turning off their panic systems, and restoring the bond between them.

When comfort is not forthcoming, both lose out on nature's analgesic, and the stress of their discomfort intensifies until something shuts it down. In the best scenario, each is able to mobilize his or her capacity for self-soothing and calm down. At worst, they give up, go numb, and fall back asleep. In 2012, professor Wendy Middlemiss and her colleagues at the University of North Texas discovered something remarkable in their study of mother-infant interactions: when a baby left to cry finally calmed down, the mother's stress (as measured by her level of the stress hormone, cortisol) dropped immediately; however, the infant's cortisol level remained high for hours afterwards.[28] It was a small study, but if further research confirms the results, then it would be safe to suggest that the quiet that follows an infant's unattended separation cries is not so much a sign of successful self-soothing as one of despair.

At present, despite pediatric support for independent sleep and formal sleep-training in the United Kingdom, the United States, Canada, and Germany, it appears that the majority of parents in these countries sleep with or near their infants at least part of the time. Regardless of the approach parents take to their babies' sleep, the bedtime battles that many have come to consider normal, and the comforting rituals and accessories that support a burgeoning baby nursery industry, seem to be necessitated by adult desires to instill their cultural values and practices despite our species' evolution in the context of shared sleep. While biology necessitates sleep, culture defines its shape and length, character and conditions.

Developing Nervous Systems

Interviews with parents from a variety of cultures reveal that many believe there is a connection between infant sleep arrangements and adult behavior. Mayan mothers, who sleep with their babies and nurse on demand, explained to researchers that these practices make their children feel close to other people and more likely to understand and learn from them. Japanese mothers sleep with their babies next to them in order to foster interdependence and group harmony, in contrast to many Northern European and American mothers, who teach their babies to sleep separately to foster independence and self-reliance.[29]

Having grown up with a room of my own from a very early age, near woods where I spent most of my free time by myself, I was used to an exceptional amount of space and privacy when I entered adulthood. So it was an adjustment, to say the least, when I decided to move into a small three-room house with my partner and her young child at age twenty-six. That was the year I grew a white streak in my hair. Much as I yearned to relieve myself of the alienation and loneliness I had always known, it was not easy to learn the art of interdependency in close quarters. Sharing my bed with another was surprisingly uncomfortable, even distressing. The very presence of another body, its weight and warmth, airs, odors, and noises, often kept me awake for hours. I usually startled when touched or bumped, and I took some time to settle back down. Even when I grew to enjoy the company of another, I slept better alone.

Now, after decades of sharing my bed with a partner, I occasionally feel small and frightened when I find myself alone. That is when I break the rules and call my dogs and cats onto the bed to nestle with me. At this point in my life, I find the pressure of a warm body curled up against the small of my back or behind my knees immensely comforting. It is a comfort that feels creaturely, as if satisfying an instinct that has persisted through aeons of evolution. While it is not literally skin-to-skin (much as my animals would like to burrow under my covers), I suspect it provides the same solace.

I remember a time when a friend was having difficulty getting her oldest daughter, then a wide-eyed and wiggly nine-month-old, down for a nap. She tried placing her in various positions, comforting her with baby talk, walking around and jiggling her softly, but nothing worked. Then her sister-in-law, who was visiting from India, offered to help. Her sister-in-law lay down on her back, placed her squirming niece on her rotund belly, began slow, deep breathing, and the two fell fast asleep.

Infants are born with immature nervous systems, dependent

upon caretakers to develop their neurological abilities to regulate their arousal levels, physiologically and psychologically. A parent's smell, touch, voice, and movements normalize the baby's breathing, body temperature, calorie absorption, stress hormone levels, immune status, and oxygenation—especially during the first year of life. Physical presence and reliable reassurance from a caregiver (including simple eye contact, holding, feeding, talking, playing, singing, and cooing) builds the neural circuitry that enables the child to calm down—and wake up—when needed.[30]

While some babies cry less, and sleep more easily, than others from the very beginning, none are born with the ability to quiet themselves down when they get upset. We develop that capacity through hundreds, even thousands, of comforting exchanges with our caregivers. Even though parents cannot always attend to their babies as quickly or adequately as they would like, due to other responsibilities, frustration, or exhaustion, infants gradually learn to trust that others can help them calm down when they cannot manage it on their own. As they grow into toddlers, they begin to develop the ability to comfort themselves alone with reminders of their caregivers—transitional objects that feel, taste, smell, or sound like them.[31] This is what constitutes self-soothing, and it relies upon neural circuitry that functions largely outside our conscious awareness and control. As any good insomniac can tell you, we cannot will ourselves to sleep. Nor can we make ourselves wide awake the next day if we have not had enough sleep.

In the burgeoning field of infant development, it is becoming increasingly clear that babies who are repeatedly left alone to cry can develop a hypersensitivity—and a reduced resilience—to stress, which remains with them for years.[32] That vulnerability can manifest in later years as a tendency toward anxiety and insomnia, or depression and oversleeping, depending upon whether the panic system got stuck in protest or despair. They may rely upon drugs, alcohol, or destructive behaviors like self-cutting to control emotional extremes. They may also have difficulty creating and sustaining supportive relationships, since our capacities for empathy, trust, and accommodation run thin when we have felt abandoned too many times.[33]

This is not to say that using some version of the Ferber method to sleep-train your baby will make him or her grow up into an anxious, uncooperative, alienated, or depressed adult. The autonomic systems that regulate arousal are put into place during our waking and sleeping hours as infants and may not necessitate co-sleeping to sustain the reliable, responsive parent-infant relationship that ensures healthy development. Every time a caretaker comforts a crying baby, the action buffers any stress sensitivity that may be accruing, cultivates empathy, and develops resilience. It may simply be a matter of responding often and quickly enough to prevent that instinctual panic system from taking over.[34]

However, cross-cultural studies have shown that children who sleep in the same room with their parents between birth and five years of age tend to be happier, less fearful, and more cooperative than their counterparts who sleep alone. As adults, they experience less anxiety and guilt, and display greater confidence, independence, and satisfaction.[35] Since these studies were unable to isolate infant sleep practices from a host of other cultural and relational factors, such as the amount of physical contact between babies and their caregivers during the day, their results should be taken with some caution. Even so, they are striking.

The very idea that the conditions of our sleep as infants, which we do not even remember, could have any correlation with our happiness as adults continues to amaze me and to fuel my desire to understand what exactly happens when we sleep.

4

SLEEP STAGES: WESTERN SCIENCE AND EASTERN PHILOSOPHY

Ever since Aristotle declared that sleep is the privation of waking life, our nightly slumber has been conceived of as the absence, or debasement, of consciousness in the West. Many considered it to be a state of dormancy when nothing much happened, revealing the Western preference for activity over stillness. Scientific reliance upon measurable phenomena made sleep even more invisible, a perceptual hole in time that defied examination. It was easy to assume that the hours we spent in bed served our need for rest and nothing else. When twentieth-century electroencephalogram (EEG) recordings of brain activity demonstrated that sleep is a remarkably active time, the shape of our slumber and its distinct phases began to appear. The discovery spawned the new field of sleep research, and labs sprung up across the country and the world to observe and record the activities of our sleeping brains. By the end of the century, new imaging techniques capable of tracking blood flow, metabolism, hormone levels, and oxygenation provided mountains of data, and scientists mined the information to construct fascinating models of what happens when we lie down and close our eyes.

Sleep is characterized by two essential features—a reduced response to outer stimulation and the ability to wake up quickly—which distinguish it from other similar states, such as coma, anesthesia, hypnosis, hibernation, or death. When the sleep switch flips on, our brains shut down (most) sensory input and reduce motor output, in effect disabling our capacity to engage with the world. The supply of brain chemicals that facilitate short-term memory and self-reflection is cut off, making it difficult to observe and remember what happens when we sleep. When we have slept long enough, the sleep switch flips off, reversing these conditions, and we open our eyes.

However, sleep is not a single, unvarying state of consciousness. It has its own fluctuations, what could be called an ongoing dialogue, between deeper and lighter phases with chemical signatures and brain wave patterns that are as different from each other as they are from waking. While other stages have been identified based on EEG patterns, they are essentially preludes and postludes to these two basic types of sleep: rapid eye movement (REM) sleep and slow-wave (SW) sleep. These two kinds of sleep alternate some five to six times a night, every ninety minutes on average, serving different, though interconnected, roles.

REM Sleep

REM, the busiest stage of sleep, was named by Nathaniel Kleitman because our eyes dart back and forth beneath closed lids and our brain waves speed up into highly differentiated flurries while our bodies lie still, temporarily paralyzed. One sleep researcher described it this way: "The brain is on fire… but the body is a cold fish."[1] REM is so active, it literally heats up the brain, requiring further stages of sleep to cool down. The sympathetic nervous system triggers bouts of rapid heartbeats, heavy or arrested breathing, spikes in blood pressure, and faster metabolism. Dreams are vivid, abundant, and easier to remember during this stage. The capacity for REM sleep is very old in evolutionary terms; one prominent sleep researcher, J. Allan Hobson, has suggested that it preceded and fostered the development of waking consciousness.[2]

While we tend to think of ourselves as unconscious when we sleep, most contemporary neuroscientists would agree with ancient philosophers that we are conscious when we dream. After all, we experience dream events as real in the moment. Neuroscientist Rodolfo Llinás went so far as to state that dreaming "is consciousness itself in the absence of input from the senses."[3] Neurologist Oliver Sacks inverted the equation to make the same point when he stated, "Waking consciousness is dreaming—but dreaming constrained by external reality."[4]

These assertions are based in part on the discovery that our brains recruit essentially the same networks of neuronal assemblies when we are awake and letting our minds wander as when we are asleep and dreaming in REM.[5] With the development of functional imaging techniques, scientists have been able to track activation patterns in the brain when people are performing tasks, daydreaming, meditating, and sleeping. Expecting to find the most activity when we are engaged in the world, scientists were surprised to discover that our brains erupt into even greater, spontaneous activity whenever we withdraw attention from the task at hand and let our minds wander.

This default mode network, which has been likened to dark matter because of its previous invisibility, evokes an intrinsic, spontaneous reverie akin to the stream of consciousness vividly portrayed by writers like Marcel Proust, James Joyce, Virginia

Woolf and William Faulkner. In *Mrs. Dalloway*, Virginia Woolf brings the reader into mind of a woman about to take her depressed husband, Septimus, to the doctor:

> She must go back again to Septimus since it was almost time for them to be going to Sir William Bradshaw. She must go back and tell him, go back to him sitting there on the green chair under the tree, talking to himself, or to that dead man Evans, whom she had only seen once for a moment in the shop. He had seemed a nice, quiet man; a great friend of Septimus's, and he had been killed in the War. But such things happen to every one. Every one has friends who were killed in the War. Everyone gives up something when they marry. She had given up her home.[6]

In default mode, when we are not attending to something or someone outside of us, we recall bits of past experiences, envision future possibilities, wonder why people behave the way they do, and ponder moral issues. In short, we exercise our imaginations. Imaginative exploration, whether expressed in the ideas of waking life or the images of dream sleep, is the brain's default mode and primary enterprise, consuming more energy than any other activity. When August Strindberg sat down to write a play based on dreams, he explained: "… the imagination spins, weaving new patterns on a flimsy basis of reality: a mixture of memories, experiences, free associations, absurdities, and improvisations. The characters split, double, multiply, evaporate, condense, dissolve, and merge."[7] The dreamer, Strindberg added, "does not judge, does not acquit, simply relates." Through it all, we concoct a self that is half remembered and half foreseen to carry us through life's challenges.

When we are awake, we know we are daydreaming because the self-reflective, reality-testing parts of our brains remain involved. Logic and narrative continue to shape our perceptions, and we hold a dual awareness of both inner fantasy and outer reality at the same time. But that changes when we fall asleep and enter REM. The prefrontal cortex, which enables us to maintain self-awareness and organize experience, goes off-line.[8] Even though lucid dreamers maintain some awareness of themselves and their surroundings while engaging in their dreams, most of us lack this ability, or the will to cultivate it. As a result, we are immersed in the internally generated worlds of our dreams unconstrained by external reality.

Dreaming may turn out to be, as the nineteenth century New England minister once observed, "an act of pure imagination." However, dream experience rarely makes sense in the logic of the waking world, and it has a way of evaporating the moment we open our eyes and become aware of our surroundings. Furthermore, it is rarely continuous or congruent with waking awareness, making it difficult to integrate into the storyline of our daily lives. The ancient Greeks acknowledged this fact by explaining that we must cross the River Lethe to leave the cave of sleep, so that the waters of forgetting can wash away our dreams before we open our eyes. To refuse the waters of forgetting and keep hold of dream reality in the outer world is to court disaster. Only the very adept, the great seers, dare take the risk.

The Deep Well of Memory

One of the most notable facts about REM sleep is that it engages the amygdala, part of the limbic system, popularly known as the emotional brain. The amygdala is responsible for our fight-or-flight reactions. Ordinarily, when we encounter a new situation, the thinking part of the brain, the cortex, considers information received from the senses before directing the limbic system to generate an emotional reaction. However, there are times when we need to act more quickly than that, especially in the face of danger, and instinct takes over. The sense of alarm triggers a shortcut in the brain, prompting the amygdala to spring into action before all the information is sorted out. In short, we jump first and look later.

The classic example given to demonstrate this effect is the way people instinctively jump away at the sight of a snake, even though it may turn out later to be a coiled rope. The reaction occurs before the visual information is fully integrated—but the error can save a life, so it has a clear evolutionary advantage. This unconscious circuitry is activated more often than we imagine, not only in situations of potential threat, but whenever we respond without thinking, which is most of the time. Every time it happens, another experience is grafted onto that emotional circuitry, forming the patterns of unconscious belief that filter our perceptions and inform our reactions. Cognitive psychologists report that these schemas, akin to what Carl Jung called complexes, shape our conscious beliefs and attitudes, including our political convictions, without our knowing.[9]

Carl Jung called his "feeling-toned complexes" the architects of our dreams, foreshadowing the discovery of amygdala involvement in REM state dreams a century later. Since we are deprived of sensory input when we sleep, it is possible that some of our dreams are little more than variations of our schemas, triggered by recent events. During REM sleep, emotionally charged events are replayed and revised without the oversight of logic, the inhibition of morals, or the intrusion of facts from our short-term memory banks. This allows a creative free play, enabling us to draw from the sum of our experiences to imaginatively correct mistakes and explore new ways of handling situations.

Psychologist and neuroscientist Antti Revonsuo and his colleagues at the University of Turku, Finland, published a seminal paper in 2000 proposing that REM sleep evolved to do just that: rehearse and adapt inherited survival strategies.[10] Noting that the vast majority of the dreams people remember involve threatening situations, they reasoned that negative dreams might function as "rehearsal for similar real events, so that threat recognition and avoidance happens faster and more automatically in comparable real situations." If so, they are like the drills athletes perform on a daily basis to perfect their skills. I hope I never have to run from a tsunami or drive downhill without brakes, but I have practiced both in my dreams.

While these what-if scenarios could prepare us for future challenges, they may also help us to undo, or redo, past ones. Evolutionary neuropsychologist and sleep researcher Patrick McNamara calls the process of learning by reimagining past events counterfactual simulation and observed that it often occurs in REM dreams.[11] "We humans do most of our everyday learning," McNamara added, "via these sorts of counterfactual simulations." For example, we may imagine or dream of telling someone something we have not been able to say in person. Both processes—Revonsuo's threat simulations and McNamara's counterfactual ones—rely upon the extraordinary human capacity to learn from experience with the help of imagination, which we have developed over millions of years of evolution.

REM sleep evolved about 130 million years ago when mammals gave up laying eggs and began to bear live young. Even though live birth increased the vulnerability of the young, it vastly enhanced their ability to learn and adapt through experience in the current environment, expanding behavioral options beyond genetically driven instincts. To this day, the more immature a newborn mammal is, the more time it spends in REM sleep translating experience into neuronal wiring. Human babies spend a full nine hours a day in REM, compared to the two hours adults spend. These and other discoveries have prompted researchers to propose that REM sleep is essential to brain plasticity, developing the nervous system by strengthening some connections and weakening others, continually rewriting the scripts by which we live our lives.[12]

This could explain why we spend so much time running, hiding, or defending ourselves from danger in our dreams—even from wild animals we have never encountered in waking life. We are rehearsing and improving our means of survival, running the maze of life in all its myriad variations, with amygdala-driven beating hearts. The most commonly reported dreams worldwide, those of encountering snakes or spiders; being lost, chased, or naked; and teeth falling out, seem to refer to a time when we lived in the wild. Carl Sagan even speculated that the most universal dream—that of falling—stems from the early days of our evolution when our ancestors slept in trees.[13]

This is an intriguing notion. The possibility sheds light on the discovery by dream researcher David Foulkes that young children dream much more of animals than adults do.[14] On the one hand, it makes sense because children are typically attracted to small creatures. There seems to be a secret affinity—even identification—between the two. On the other hand, little kids are surrounded and cared for by people, and one would think they would dream more about them. But they do not; they do not even dream about themselves.

Instead, their night worlds are largely inhabited by animals, not the pets they live with so much as the bears, sharks, and snakes that populate fairy tales. It would be easy to assume that children's books and movies supply the animal characters for their dream lives, and they might to some extent. However, one could also argue that children's stories are filled with thinking, feeling, and talking mammals because kids respond more to them than to human characters. Having less experience in life, small children may identify more with animals because they are closer to our creaturely origins.

I was prone to fevers as a young child, and I remember having the same dream every time: elephants were stampeding, and I could see their mammoth feet pounding the dirt, spewing clouds of dust. I was watching from ground level, as if I were hiding behind a bush. I have no idea where the scenario came from, as we did not have television and rarely went to movies. I had probably seen a lonely elephant or two at the zoo, but the sight and sound of that stampede must have come from somewhere else.

There are times when our dreams seem to draw from a well of memory so deep that we cannot see the bottom, one that is fed by our personal experiences within familial and cultural histories. Maybe there is something like genetic memory accessible in sleep. After all, our bodies have physical traits left over from our animal ancestry. The coccyx at the base of the spine is considered to be the remnant of a tail, and the reflex of goose bumps remains from when we had fur and raised our hackles.

Slow-Wave Sleep

At the other extreme from REM sleep is slow-wave (SW) sleep, a deep, nearly inaccessible slumber that is characterized by slow, high-amplitude, synchronized brain waves. It appears to be the most restorative form of sleep, regenerating tissues, building bones and muscles, and strengthening immunity, all of which are facilitated by the release of growth hormones and a reduction in cortisol levels. SW sleep also burns fat and maintains cardiovascular health, which explains why sleep deprivation contributes to the development of obesity and heart problems. It is hard to wake people from SW sleep, and even when successful, they usually remain groggy (and grumpy!) for some time.

The calming, parasympathetic branch of the autonomic nervous system predominates in SW sleep, reducing metabolism, blood pressure, and heart and breath rates. Even so, SW sleep is the source of our most disturbing and dangerous sleep disorders—night terrors and sleepwalking—perhaps because we are so far from consciousness. SW sleep constitutes less than one-quarter of our time asleep, but it dominates the first few hours and replenishes itself faster than any other kind of sleep. It seems to be the most necessary stage of sleep. Though dreaming occurs in SW sleep, it tends to be more fragmentary, vague, and thought-like.

One of the most intriguing features of deep, SW sleep is that the brain's default mode that springs into action whenever our minds wander and dream ceases to function properly.[15] This important, intrinsic brain function operates throughout all the other phases of waking and sleeping life—even when we go under anesthesia—but the connections weaken in our deepest, most restorative sleep. It appears that when we drop into SW sleep, the persistent mental chatter we live with day in and day out, what Buddhists call the monkey mind, grinds to a halt. With it goes that strong sense of self we maintain to organize and consolidate our experiences. It is as if our minds finally empty out and stop imagining reality.

Curiously, the amount of SW sleep we get decreases dramatically over the human lifespan.[16] While SW sleep constitutes nearly 20 percent of our nightly slumber in young adulthood, it is only 3 percent by midlife. Up to one-quarter of fifty-year-olds have no

SW sleep, and this percentage increases with age. Because growth hormones are secreted only during SW sleep, a reduction in deep sleep also lowers the levels of these hormones. The combination can account for many features of the aging process, including loss of muscle tone and physical strength, increased body fat, thinning of the skin, fatigue, diminished sexual desire, memory loss, and immune malfunction. No wonder the Irish say sleep is better than medicine. It would not be an exaggeration to say that SW sleep is critical to our nightly restoration and healthy aging.

SW sleep, and its polar opposite, REM sleep, have been defined and described in detail by scientists around the world using advanced technologies to measure everything from brain wave frequencies to hormonal levels. I was surprised to discover that ancient philosophers, primarily from Eastern traditions, developed a parallel body of knowledge about sleep by carefully observing and recording subjective experiences. Their accounts are remarkably congruent with those developed by contemporary scientists, despite the different tools they employed to elucidate the secret life of sleep.

Eastern Philosophical Perspectives

When the religious scholar Huston Smith asked Indian philosopher Dr. T. M. P. Mahadevan to describe the difference between Eastern and Western thought, Mahadevan answered that Westerners philosophize from a single state of consciousness, the waking state, whereas East Indians draw from all states of consciousness, including those of sleep, to develop their views of reality. Ancient Hindu, Buddhist, Taoist, and Sufi teachings derive from thousands of years of close observation of the full range of conscious and unconscious human experience and, similar to those of Western scientists, their texts make distinctions between deep and dream sleep.[17]

The earliest Hindu philosophical texts, the *Upanishads*, which date back before the sixth century BC, describe three basic states or stages of experience—waking, dreaming, deep sleep—and a final, transcendent state that encompasses and moves beyond the first three. The famous Sanskrit word *aum* (also spelled as *ohm* and *om*) known to most meditators, is written with curved lines that represent these four states of consciousness.[18] As we move through the first three in the course of a day, we gradually shift our awareness from physical objects outside of us (during waking life) to awareness of object impressions within us (dreaming life) to the absence of any awareness of sense objects (deep sleep) and back up again.[19] In the second state, dreaming, the *Upanishads* state that the sleeping individual "projects from himself chariots, spans, roads. There are no blisses there, no pleasures, no delights. But he projects from himself blisses, pleasures, delights… For he is a creator." The texts appear to view dreaming as a creative power, a form of imaginative play, which disappears when we drop into dreamless sleep, the third stage of consciousness. Dreamless sleep is described as a blissful place with no sensory awareness, no witness, and no desire—the closest thing to enlightenment we can experience.

Buddhism, which originated in Hindu India, similarly values deep sleep over dreaming as an opportunity to experience the Clear Light Mind, a transparent awareness that is unobstructed by habitual attitudes and beliefs derived from past experiences. Buddhism teaches that these habits of mind cloud our awareness by day and spawn our dreams by night, generating endless, entangling dramas. Noting that dreams vanish upon waking, just as bubbles burst and frost evaporates in the first light of day, Buddhists remind us that everything is ultimately insubstantial and impermanent.[20] In short, they are imaginary.

Tibetan Buddhists further state that the processes of sleeping, dreaming, and waking we undergo every twenty-four hours so resemble those of dying, passing through an intermediate state called the *bardo*, and being reborn into a new life that we can consider them a daily rehearsal. Deep, dreamless sleep is one of the few opportunities to escape our ephemeral entanglements and wake up to the eternal peace of radiant emptiness. Characteristically, the Taoist proverb puts it more simply: "Sleep is the intelligence of not knowing anything."

Sufism, the mystical branch of Islam, outlines similar stages of consciousness but with a few differences.[21] The dreaming state, *Malkut*, is understood to exist when we are asleep *and* when we are awake and absorbed in our imaginations, what contemporary neuroscientists would call the brain's default mode. In both cases, the emotional residues of our days are gathered and clothed in images, those of our nighttime dreams and our daytime fantasies. Thinkers, artists, seers, and sages gain insight and inspiration from this state. However, we occupy it much more than we realize, and we easily confuse our creative dreaming with reality. Sufism asserts that anything outside the present moment is a dream. Whenever we remember the past or imagine the future, we are dreaming, spinning worlds out of our own creative powers, fashioning our own heavens and hells.

When Sufis speak of waking up, they are referring to turning attention away from the creative play of dreaming to the peace and stillness of deep sleep, known as Lahut. In Lahut, we return to our essential unlimited natures in communion with the divine. The conditions of our waking lives no longer exist, and all our sufferings, agitations, and exhaustion are washed away. The thirteenth-century Persian poet, jurist, and Sufi mystic Jalal ad-Din Rumi described the experience in his famous poem "Sleep of the Body the Soul's Awakening":

Every night Thou freest our spirits from the body
And its snare, making them pure as rased tablets.
Every night spirits are released from this cage,
And set free, neither lording it nor lorded over.
At night prisoners are unaware of their prison,
At night kings are unaware of their majesty.
Then there is no thought or care for loss or gain,
No regard to such an one or such an one.[22]

The Clear Light of Deep Sleep

We may not remember that place of peace in the morning, but I believe we can see it in the faces of those deeply asleep. There is an almost angelic look to those calm countenances. I remember the amazement I felt as a child the first time I saw the mean older sister of a friend sleeping early one morning, curled up on her side in bed, hair strewn across the pillow, her hand in a baby's fist next to her cheek. She was unbelievably beautiful. Since that time, I have tried to find a sleeping face that did not seem precious to me, to no avail.

When our facial muscles relax, the masks we create to make our ways in the world disappear. Stripped of our socially constructed selves, we seem to revert to an essential creaturely nature, which is neither good nor bad but strangely innocent. The sight inevitably evokes sympathy in me, regardless of the person's actions in waking life. Perhaps it is a biological instinct, like the one that responds to the large, widely set eyes of babies, to protect the vulnerable amidst us.

Occasionally, especially when waking slowly, I have been aware of an astonishing absence of the anxieties that accompany me by day. I first noticed this after a friend of mine committed suicide in my second year of college. For days, weeks, and months afterward, I would wake up as usual, and then suddenly remember her death like a punch to my solar plexus, plunging me into agonizing grief. But for those few moments while I was coming to, I was without suffering, as if coming from a place where her death either never occurred or was assimilated in a way that did not cause me anguish, a place of peaceful emptiness.

Marcel Proust described it well in *Remembrance of Things Past*: "From those profound slumbers, we awake in a dawn, not knowing who we are, being nobody, newly born, ready for anything, the brain emptied of that past which was life until then." Sleep was the only time that awful year I could lay down my load, forget everything, and be forgotten, even if the next morning, or next nightmare, threw me back in the ring.

Proust added that "deep slumber" opens us to "all the mysteries which we imagine ourselves not to know… and into which we are in reality initiated almost every night." Every now and then, I wake from sleep with a phrase repeating in my mind that feels utterly momentous. Sometimes I see it written out; at other times, I hear it like a voice-over in a movie, or I just know it. Whichever way, I have the sense that I have emerged from a sacred realm with an answer to the world's problems, and I scribble it down immediately so I will not forget it.

Inevitably, though, when I return the next day to ponder the words I have written, they seem to have shriveled up into silliness, obscurity, or downright nonsense overnight. For example, one night before a difficult day at work, I woke up with these words on my mind: "Compassion is the ability to hold dear." At the time, I felt lifted into my day by this reminder of the true nature of caring. Now, I am embarrassed to write the words down because they sound like a saying from a Hallmark card. I suspect that revelations like this that are so vulnerable to waking diminishment come from the depths of sleep, where dreaming is typically less visual and more declarative. Perhaps they are residues of the clear light that Buddhists describe. Whatever the case, these rare occurrences feel like small blessings.

These occasional revelations also leave me wondering, at times, if the world that spawns them somewhere in the watery depths of my sleep is actually the real world and my waking one is just the dusty froth that blows across its surface. Sufi teacher Hazrat Inayat Khan suggested this might be the case, explaining: "We do not realize that, when we are awake, we are covering ourselves from another world which, in fact, is more real... When we cover ourselves from what is more real, we say, 'I am awake' and, when we cover ourselves from what is unreal and illusion, we say we are asleep."

This is the mystic's vision. No wonder Hindu, Sufi, and Buddhist practitioners seek to bring the clear light from deep sleep into conscious daily life. It is not easy, as the worlds are virtually incomprehensible to each other. While scientists investigate and theorize about the mechanics of forgetting upon waking, the chemical shifts that enable one kind of awareness and disable another, it may just be that language, being linear and conceptual, simply cannot express the ephemeral and imagistic complexities of such deep experiences.

But the difficulties of carrying something from deep sleep into waking awareness have not kept people from trying. For over two thousand years, Hindu yogis have trained themselves to go straight into deep sleep, a place conceived of as communion with the divine beyond space and time as we know them, and skip or skim over dreaming in order to keep hold of their deepest awareness when waking. Their practices, known as Yoga Nidra, derived from the *Mandukya Upanishad*, are still taught today.[23] Taoist teachers recommended meditations, cleansing practices, sleeping positions, and diets to cultivate the inner peace and clarity (the "luminous pearl") that allowed them to shorten time spent dreaming and stay longer in deep, dreamless sleep. For nearly as long, Chinese Taoists and Tibetan Buddhists have practiced dream yoga, learning to dispel fears, transform content, and recognize the ever-changing nature of life while dreaming and later, in waking life.[24] Both cultivate meditative states that can best be understood as hybrids of sleeping and waking awareness, reminding us that the two are not so different. As Hazrat Inayat Khan explained: "In reality, sleep and the wakeful state are nothing but the turning of the consciousness from one side to the other."

When sleeping awareness and waking awareness overlap, as they do when we wake in the midst of a long night of sleep, we have the unique opportunity to witness that turning of consciousness apart from the glare of daytime demands and under the spell of darkness. Midnight wakings are as distinct from daytime wakefulness as they are from sleep itself.

5

BETWEEN SLEEPS: THE MIDNIGHT WATCH

Imagine volunteering for a study in which you would spend every night in a windowless dark room for fourteen hours for an entire month. There would be no sources of light—no matches, lamps, televisions, or computers—just a deep, flawless dark for fourteen hours. Our prehistoric ancestors in the higher latitudes lived under these conditions every winter before the advent of artificial light, but now in the twenty-first century, few of us have had the experience. Even campers build fires and carry flashlights. It is next to impossible to escape the light that pervades our days and invades our nights.

Like Brooding Hens

Psychiatrist Thomas A. Wehr, a sleep researcher with the National Institute of Mental Health, secured eight student volunteers for this experiment in the early 1990s.[1] At first, the volunteers slept an average of eleven hours a night, nearly the entire period of darkness, probably catching up on lost sleep. After a few weeks, they settled into an average of nearly nine spread out over a period of twelve hours, with a few hours of peaceful wakefulness in the middle. Their early evening sleep was primarily deep SW sleep, and the morning one was characterized by the dreams that come with REM sleep. It also took the students one to two hours to fall asleep, something few of us would tolerate nowadays.

When I first read about Wehr's experiment, I imagined that the volunteers could not wait for the month to be over, having had to lie around doing nothing for so long. Not true. Many later reported missing the "quiet wakefulness" of the mid-night hours between sleeps, what early American novelist Nathaniel Hawthorne called "an intermediate space, where the business of life does not intrude; where the passing moment lingers, and becomes truly the present." Wehr, who monitored his subjects day and night, described this time as a "quiescent, meditative state" with an endocrinology all its own. It was an inwardly focused space unlike ordinary daytime wakefulness, one in which it was easy to wonder, muse, and ponder. "It is tempting to speculate," Wehr added, "that in prehistoric times this arrangement provided a channel of communication between dreams and waking life that has gradually been closed off as humans have compressed and consolidated their sleep."

He also noted that volunteers had high levels of the pituitary hormones prolactin and melatonin throughout their long nights. Prolactin and melatonin promote a restful calm and satisfaction, enabling broody hens, nursing mothers (and nurturing fathers) to sit quietly for long periods of time. It gives them that dreamy, dazed, contented look I have often envied, as if all is right with the world, and they are doing exactly what they should be doing. Prolactin also promotes neurogenesis, the process by which new nerve cells are generated. By day, the students reported feeling more awake than ever. Wehr tested them, using a standard daytime sleepiness scale, and found out that not only did they "feel more awake, they were more awake." When the study was over, and the students returned to their regular schedules of one long sleep a day, their melatonin levels dropped off and prolactin levels did not sustain through the night. With these changes went, I suspect, the capacity for calm, dream-informed rest and contentment.

It may be that sleep is naturally interspersed with wakefulness when circumstances allow it. The one time in my adult life when I had no work or school schedule to organize my days and nights, and I lived outside in rural Oklahoma for a month, I quickly fell into napping through the heat of the day and staying awake for chunks of the night, listening to the stirrings of nocturnal creatures, watching the stars turn slowly overhead, drifting in and out of dreams. Comparative literature also suggests that this pattern of sleeping more than once over twenty-four hours is the rule, rather than the exception, throughout the animal kingdom and among preindustrial peoples. In northern climates with long dark winters, both periods of sleep tend to occur at night, as they did in Wehr's study. In warmer climates, a midday siesta replaces the first sleep. When researching sleep patterns in premodern Europe, historian Roger Ekirch found frequent references to the "first sleep" or "deep sleep" and the "second sleep" or "morning sleep," and the "watch" between them.[2]

SW sleep dominates the first half of the night, and unless we are unduly agitated by the events of the previous day, or worried about the one to come, mid-night spells of wakefulness can be remarkably peaceful, as if colored by the quiet, deep sleep that preceded it. People prone to such awakenings often read for a while, ponder a dream, or simply listen to the wind outside. Henry David Thoreau used to place a pen and a blank piece of paper under his pillow every night, and if he woke, he would write in the dark. Writer Brian W. Aldiss described the lucidity of these hours: "It's at night, when perhaps we should be dreaming, that the mind is most clear, that we are most able to hold all our life in the palm of our skull." According to the *Buddhacarita*, a second-century poetic saga of Buddha's life, Buddha received his enlightenment during several night watches.[3] Having destroyed disturbances of the mind, and attained mental concentration, Buddha remembered his past lives as if living them over again during the first watch. On the second watch, he saw the workings of karma and reincarnation, and finally achieved enlightenment on the fourth watch of the night. Though the tale may be apocryphal, it speaks to an ancient understanding of the revelatory power that occasionally arrives between sleeps.

When artificial light entered our nights and industrialization commandeered our days, we achieved the capacity to remain active and productive regardless of the time of day or night. The borders of darkness no longer curtailed our lives, and we filled our hours with activity of one kind or another. By the eighteenth century, London's coffeehouses and pleasure gardens were thronged with visitors all night, fueled by the influx of imported coffee and sugar.[4] In the twenty-first century, the demands of round-the-clock commerce and accessibility continually turn our attention to the outside world at the expense of our private inner lives. By forgoing our historical habit of mid-night waking in order to consolidate and shorten our sleep time, we may have lost our taste for restful reflection, dream awareness, and the pleasures of nocturnal life.

Now, when people wake for one or two hours at night, they are apt to call it insomnia and ask their doctors for sleeping pills. The NSF's 2008 Sleep in America Poll reported that 35 percent of Americans said they wake up in the middle of the night three or more times a week, and of those who woke, 43 percent had a hard time falling back asleep.[5] Variously called middle-of-the-night insomnia, sleep maintenance insomnia, or simply middle insomnia, periods of wakefulness at night make up the most common type of insomnia—if it is even appropriate to use that label. "An alternative explanation," noted Wehr, "could be that a natural pattern of human sleep is breaking through into an artificial world in which it seems unfamiliar and unwelcome."[6]

One of the interesting facts about aging is that sleep tends to become more broken, as if reverting back to this ancient pattern. By age fifty, many women and men are up in the night for a while, much to the annoyance and frustration of those who maintain demanding work and family lives by day. People in their seventies and eighties often slip into an afternoon nap to make up for the loss.[7] As a result, the elderly spend more time between waking and sleeping, which could contribute to the confusion that often accompanies our later years but may also allow more time for the interior activities of reflection and imagination. When a friend of mine in his early eighties heard that I was working on a book about sleep, he told me that he sleeps less as he gets older but spends more and more time in quiet contemplation. He considers it a spiritual practice required by the conditions of aging, including the reduction of sleep.

Ever since I learned about Wehr's study and Ekirch's historical confirmation, I have tried to approach my nocturnal waking hours with a different attitude. About once a week, I wake when it is still deeply dark and the house is quiet except for the snores of the animals. Once my eyes are open and I become aware of my surroundings, it is an hour or two before sleep finds me again. I inevitably start worrying that I will not get enough sleep, and I imagine what miseries would come of it the next day. Years ago, in the middle of the night, I convinced myself that I had pancreatic cancer because I felt an unusual pain in my abdomen. Author

Blake Butler, a chronic insomniac, calls the tendency to do this sleep catastrophizing.[8] Anxiety only fuels insomnia. It makes the clock tick louder and turns a few hours into an eternity. The harder I try to sleep, the worse it gets, as I flop from side to side with frustrated sighs and furtive glances at the clock.

One of the cruelties of insomnia is that the effort to escape ensures its failure because there's a part of our brains that keeps checking to see if we are accomplishing our aims, thereby keeping us awake. It is the same part that makes it impossible not to think about something, like the proverbial pink elephant. The more we try not to think of the pink elephant, or not to stay awake, the more likely we will. It is a vicious cycle, a losing battle. We might as well give up, let go of our distress over being awake, and see what happens. After all, our expectations of falling asleep quickly and sleeping through seven or eight hours may simply be artifacts of chronic sleep deprivation and artificial light, as Wehr came to believe.[9]

Now, when I wake in the night, I tell myself that repose is still rest and it is a gift to get a few extra hours when I do not have to do anything or be responsible to anyone. The French call this place of semiconscious inactivity *dorveille*, meaning "twixt sleep and wake," and many poets consider it to be the best time to write. Writer Lisa Russ Spaar explained: "As a poet, I like... that liminal space between sleep and waking, where 'reality' and inner vision blur, and all the big questions loom with heightened clarity."[10]

I try to remind myself of the Taoist instruction that sleep must be honored and entered into with respect, not as a collapse of wakefulness or a giving in to exhaustion. I call forth the image of our chickens ambling drowsily into the hen house at dusk, clucking softly as if passing the last few bits of gossip before bed, and I try to relax into that creaturely space of inattentive drifting between the shores of waking and sleeping worlds. Sometimes I throw out a topic to ponder, like flinging a stone into water, and watch what unfolds. I might consider a dream image, start a letter in my mind, or remember what it was like to sit in the shallow waters of the Caribbean, and then, inevitably, lose track of what I was doing. The next thing I know, I'm waking up to another day.

I am fortunate, however, because I usually fall back asleep. Many cannot return to sleep, and they spend hours lying awake in bed every night, or they get up and start doing things, having to drag themselves through yet another day without nearly enough shut-eye. The question of why some can drift in that mid-night peace, while others rev up into a frenzy of too much wakefulness remains an open and pressing question.

6

WHEN SLEEP NEVER COMES: INSOMNIA'S TOLL

Insomnia, which could be loosely described as difficulty sleeping, is hardly new. Nor is it restricted to Western or modernized cultures. Ancient medical texts from China to Greece give considerable attention to the problem, and it is probably safe to assume their patients asked for that help. Folk remedies, be they valerian tea, mandrake and lettuce juice poultices, back rubs, warm baths, or hot toddies, have been passed down for generations throughout the world. When I visited relatives in India several years ago, they showed me a sacred herb growing in a small pot on a pedestal in the center of their family compound courtyard; it was tulsi, otherwise known as holy basil, which has been grown for a variety of medicinal purposes, including improving sleep, for centuries. A friend of mine rubs a spot on the foreheads of her children whenever they cannot sleep, something her mother and grandmother taught her, and she swears it always works.

Up to thirty-seven percent of UK adults report difficulty sleeping on most nights,[1] which strikes me as ironic, considering that we are born with the ability and practice it incessantly the first few years of life. As we grow up and grow older, a variety of forces converge to turn the natural knack for sleep into a fragile, uneasy accomplishment. Our bodies change physiologically, continually altering the amount of sleep we need, the kind we get, and the time of day we are best able to get it as we progress through the life cycle. We assume and relinquish many responsibilities, encounter differing environmental conditions, and make lifestyle choices that impact when, where, and whether we can sleep. Sleep carries us into and out of life; but in between, it seems to abandon us.

In the fourteenth century, when Mongol tribes swept down from the steppes of Central Asia and slaughtered more than thirty million people throughout Eurasia, a young Chinese refugee retreated to the mountains. Wen-siang wandered for years, bedding down in caves, ravines, and abandoned huts; subsisting on wild plants and berries; and writing poetry when he could not sleep. While many of his poems refer to sleepless nights, this one offers a particularly poignant description:

> It's a quiet night,
> but I'm not getting to sleep…
> The west wind is noisier yet;
> myriad openings hit the same note.
> Even the crickets feel sad,
> chirping under the floor…
> I wander back and forth, uneasy in mind.
> My heartbreak cannot be told;
> Silently, useless anguish fills me."[2]

Wen-siang may have been one of that small percentage of people who just are not wired to sleep, but any one of the harsh elements he encountered could have filled his nights with useless anguish: cold, hunger, pain, illness, vermin, the trials and terrors of wartime, and—the only one he mentions here—heartache. It is understandable why sleep evaded him so often. Eight centuries later, 10 to 15 percent of the general population have chronic insomnia,[3] and a solid majority admit they would rather get a good night's sleep than have sex.[4] Even children do not get the sleep they need. In 2013, researchers at Boston College published the results of an international comparison of nine- to ten-year-old students taking maths, science, and reading tests.[5] They found that 73 percent of the American students were sleep deprived, more than in any other country, although New Zealand, Saudi Arabia, Kuwait, Australia, Turkey, England, Chile, Ireland, and Finland were close behind.

While insomnia has troubled humankind for millennia, its prevalence and chronicity may be a relatively new phenomenon. The comparison begs the question: what are the conditions that hamper sleep for so many in the twenty-first century?

Don't Rest. Don't Sleep. Close the Deal.

Benjamin Franklin once famously declared: "There will be sleeping enough in the grave." Whenever I hear that quote, I imagine it was followed by something like: "So get to work, you slackers!" Franklin wanted Americans to be industrious and hardworking, if only to convince the British that they could build and run a country. His other legendary line of advice—"plough deep while sluggards sleep, and you shall have corn to sell and keep"—clearly reflected the work ethic of his Puritan ancestors, who settled the eastern seaboard and came to dominate American political and business life for the next two hundred years. Centuries later, the West has new proverbs to convince us that sleep is a form of laziness we cannot afford if we are to succeed—"You snooze, you lose" and "The best don't rest"—but they mean the same thing.

A study commissioned by Travelodge in 2013 reported that adults in the UK sleep on average just six hours and twenty-seven minutes a night, with three in five people sleeping for less than they did a year earlier. Sleep deprivation is not only affecting Britons' welfare but is also hitting the economy too, as over a fifth of adults surveyed reported they had pulled a one-day "sickie" for work over the last 12 months due to being up the night before stressed about work. On average, banking workers were getting just five hours and fifty minutes shut-eye every night. Of the industries and professions polled, public sector workers were also among the most likely to be kept awake by work anxiety. With cuts to the public sector coming on top of pay freezes and pension cuts, it comes as little surprise to find teachers, nurses and public servants dominating the list of worst-sleeping professions.[6] In this era of high unemployment, bulging workloads, shifting schedules, union busting, and corporate downsizing, many feel they have no choice but to burn the candle at both ends.

Extending light into our night times only exacerbates the problem. Because our eyes are evolutionarily programmed to use the coming and going of daylight to set our body clocks and regulate our sleep-wake cycles, nighttime light can confuse things. Ordinarily, when light receptors in our eyes perceive the onset of darkness, they signal the pineal gland to release melatonin to induce sleepiness and initiate the changes in body temperature, immunity, hunger, thirst, and arousal that accompany falling asleep. Melatonin has been called the Dracula of hormones because it only comes out at dark. The problem is that artificial light impedes the release of melatonin, making it harder to fall and stay asleep. Charles Czeisler, professor of sleep medicine at Harvard, explained: "Light affects our circadian rhythms more powerfully than any drug."[7]

In 1905, when electric street lights had already arrived to illuminate most city streets at night, Sir James Crichton-Browne, a British expert studying children's sleep, decried: "This is a sleepless age and more and more… we are turning night into day." If we were still burning candles or using gas or kerosene lanterns to see by night, it would not be such a problem because their light is dimmer, primarily in the red-orange spectrum. Even the early incandescent lightbulbs cast a yellow circle of light that did not interfere with melatonin production. However, research suggests that the blue light favored by our newer, more efficient lightbulbs and the LED screens on our electronic devices slows the release of melatonin.[8] As a result, we are apt to feel alert longer, stay up later, and get less sleep. Even though Wen-siang lived with cold, hunger, and the terrors of wartime, he had dark nights and freedom from adverse work schedules, which most in the modern world do not.

The Smoking Gun of the Modern Age

Innumerable studies have documented the ill effects of insufficient sleep, defined as getting less sleep than we need to be at our best.[9]Beyond the tiredness, fogginess, and grumpiness we commonly note the next day, less-than-optimum sleep impairs focus, judgment, problem solving, and memory. The international survey of elementary students mentioned previously confirmed what sleep scientists have predicted for years: on average, pupils who got sufficient sleep before taking their exams did better, regardless of what kind of preparation they had received.[10] Insufficient sleep slows thinking and reaction times, increasing the chance of accidents.[11] It lowers tolerance for frustration and heightens interpersonal sensitivity, making us more likely to fly off the handle over small slights, which may explain why children who do not get enough sleep are often misdiagnosed with attention deficit hyperactivity disorder (ADHD).[12]

Early studies of insufficient sleep focused on these cognitive and behavioral effects. However, research conducted since the turn of the century has made it increasingly clear that sleep loss affects our bodies as much as our brains. In 1999, Karine Speigel at the University of Brussels and Eve Van Cauter at the University of Chicago published a landmark study demonstrating that partial sleep deprivation (four hours of sleep for two nights) increased cortisol levels and reduced glucose tolerance.[13] Subsequent research indicated that sleep loss (four hours for six nights) altered the levels of hormones that regulate hunger, causing an increase in appetite and a preference for calorie-dense, high-carbohydrate foods, including sweets, salty snacks, and starchy foods.[14] Think of what you eat when you have to pull an all-nighter. Pizza? Coffee and doughnuts? I lived on brownies when I was caring for my dying father.

If insufficient sleep can cause such serious problems, what constitutes enough sleep? Over the years, experts have offered a variety of answers and reasons for the hours we require, often generalizing from common practice or personal observation, like the English proverb that recommends "six hours' sleep for a man, seven for a woman, and eight for a fool." Now sleep scientists are more circumspect, offering ranges to accommodate individual variation. At present, the Centers for Disease Control and Prevention (CDC) recommend that adolescents get eight and a half hours and adults get seven to nine, based on studies of how they perform the next day.[15] However, longevity studies reveal that people who sleep more than seven and a half hours don't live as long as those who sleep only seven hours.[16]

Some authorities avoid the numbers trap by suggesting that

if you can wake up without an alarm clock, you are getting enough sleep. However, their advice does not consider the fact that many people keep work and school schedules that do not jibe with their internal sleep-wake cycles, requiring the use of alarm clocks. Others say that if you do not get sleepy during the day, then you are probably getting enough sleep; however, the vast majority of North Americans and Europeans consume caffeinated drinks by day, so most are unable to tell if drowsiness is around the corner. To complicate matters, researchers have also discovered that a small percentage of people are long sleepers requiring nine hours, or short sleepers, who need only four or five to function well.[17] Much as we might like clear guidelines, we may have to rely on our own experiences to arrive at what works best for us as individuals.

While the quantity of sleep we get is clearly important, the quality is just as necessary to our physical, mental, and emotional well-being. Poor or fragmented sleep, which involves numerous imperceptible arousals that reduce restorative SW sleep, typically leave people feeling just as tired in the morning as when they went to bed, and it results in the same cognitive, behavioral, and metabolic problems seen with sleep deprivation. It is estimated that up to one-third of adults experience fragmented sleep. The most common causes are disrupted breathing (especially asthma and apnea), restless legs, depression, and aging, though environmental stimuli and autonomic arousal are also implicated.[18] Many of the symptoms associated with aging, from memory loss to wrinkled skin, can be attributed to reductions in SW sleep that accompany fragmented sleep. I used to wonder, as a child, why "old people" were always asking each other how they slept; now I know.

When we add caffeine to the mix, the task of defining adequate quantity and quality of sleep becomes even more complicated.

Coffee boosts confidence. It does so by increasing levels of dopamine, enhancing pleasure, alertness, and drive—just what we need to be successful in the contemporary global economy. However, it also blocks the ability of adenosine to slow us down with fatigue and drowsiness after long hours of waking activity, masking our tiredness. Neurons fire more rather than less, prompting the pituitary gland to trigger the release of adrenaline, the fight-or-flight hormone. Adrenaline speeds up our heart rates, slows digestion, and tightens muscles to prepare for the emergency. After six or seven hours, when the caffeine wears off, we feel exhausted and depressed, which leads us to… yet another cup.[19] Over time, we sleep less, and less deeply, forgoing many of the restorative functions of our nightly slumber.

While some people do better than others on short sleep, those who believe they do great on four or five hours usually do not. They just think so because sleep deprivation impairs judgment.[20] These facts alone make me want to ask presidential candidates how they sleep. In December 2008, when CNN anchor Anjali Rao asked former president Bill Clinton if he had any advice for incoming President Obama, he answered: "In my long political career, most of the mistakes I made, I made when I was too tired, because I tried too hard and worked too hard. You make better decisions when you're not too tired."[21]

Sleep Bulimia

Occasional insomnia is not a serious problem because our bodies do their best to make it up as quickly as possible, to snatch extra winks during afternoon naps, restful weekends, sick days, and vacations, often shortening the time spent in light sleep to get more of the restorative deep and dream phases of sleep. However, several consecutive nights without enough sleep can begin to wreak havoc, especially for those who ordinarily get enough. Studies have demonstrated that a week of sleeping four to five hours a night induces a cognitive impairment equivalent to a blood alcohol level of 1 percent.[22] Performance suffers, immunity weakens, stress hormones increase, and our abilities to learn, assess situations, and respond flexibly are reduced. Behind the wheel, or as a leader of a country, we become a danger to others.

The average British adult gets around 6.5 hours sleep on weeknights, an hour and a half less than they most likely need.[23] Scientists call the difference between the amount of sleep we need to feel refreshed and the amount we actually get before the alarm goes off sleep debt. That debt accumulates night after night, and at some point, it has to be repaid. As a general rule, every hour lost must be added later. Most people, myself included, try to catch up on weekends. It is a binge-and-purge habit that psychiatrist and sleep researcher Robert Stickgold has termed sleep bulimia.[24] The catch is that it does not usually work. We may feel better for a few hours on Saturday or Sunday after a long sleep the night before, but come evening, we are still impaired and more apt to make mistakes, have accidents, and overreact because the entire debt has not been repaid. To recoup fully, we need to sleep longer for several consecutive nights, something that is out of reach for many.

I learned that lesson the hard way, as I often do. When I worked as a baker in Austin, Texas, in my twenties, I started at four in the morning in order to get the croissants, breads, and cakes ready for the pre-workday rush. I would set my clock for 3:45 AM, sleep in my work clothes, flip on the light the moment the alarm rang, hop out of bed, brush my teeth, jump on my bike, and ride the mile or so down to the bakery, where I grabbed a cup of coffee and a day-old bear claw and started rolling dough. I worked until 2 PM, rode my bike to a nearby pool where I swam a mile to cool off, then rode back home for a big salad. Things would have been fine if I went to bed after that, but I did not. I had a social life, friends to visit, classes to take, meetings to attend, movies to see, and bands to hear, so I rarely made it to bed before ten or eleven. On my "weekends" (usually Monday and Tuesday) I slept in, sometimes through an entire day and night, but never really caught up on my lost sleep.

These years were happy, productive ones. It was not that I did not like to sleep; I just had so much I wanted to do and not enough time to do it. Rather than miss a party, I would dance until my legs gave way and I dropped to the floor, curled up into a ball, and fell asleep in the middle of the dance floor. Some ten years later, the pendulum swung to the other side. I collapsed, got sick, could not get well, and slept ten to twelve hours every night with a few more daytime rests. I just could not stay upright for any length of time. The way I think of it, I pulled the rubber band of my sleep purge so far, it snapped, and I had to pay the price.

Teenagers, who are perhaps the most sleep-deprived age group in our society, tend to binge and purge like there is no tomorrow. Night owls by nature, most adolescents would stay up late and sleep in if schools didn't intervene to make them get up early. According to a study in the United States, approximately 90 percent of teens do not get enough sleep.[25] They drag themselves through their days like walking zombies, often too sleepy to pay attention at school and too irritable to get along with others. Grades dip, moods plummet, fights break out, and the desire for fatty foods increases. By the time the weekend rolls around, teenagers are, on average, ten hours behind on their sleep, which may explain the stupid decisions that get made on Friday nights. Weekends and school vacations provide opportunities to begin catching up, but those twelve-to-twenty-hour slumbers for which teenagers are famous usually do not fully make up for what was lost.

Evidence of the effects of long-term sleep deprivation has been emerging, and the news is not good. Chronic sleep loss puts people at greater risk for obesity, diabetes, heart disease, strokes, mood disorders, accidents, and death.[26] It further reduces immunity and increases sensitivity to pain.[27] In light of this research, pioneering sleep scientist William Dement declared: "Sleep is one of the most important predictors of how long you will live—as important as whether you smoke, exercise, or have high blood pressure or cholesterol... Unhealthy sleep remains [our] largest, deadliest, most costly, and least studied health problem."[28]

A Brief History of Sleep Worry

Dire warnings like these strike fear into the hearts of almost everyone I know who struggles to get enough sleep. While the research is intended to inform and motivate us to improve our slumber (as if that were easy), my friends tell me that having the knowledge that losing sleep can make them fat, dumb, and reckless tortures them mercilessly when they lie awake at night, only making matters worse. Worry aggravates insomnia, often stretching minutes of blurry-eyed wakefulness into hours and entire nights.

This condition is so common, it has a medical name: psychophysiological insomnia, meaning that the physical symptoms of insomnia are fueled by psychological anxieties in a self-perpetuating cycle. I think the term tells us more about the difficulty medicine has in addressing interactions between our bodies and minds than it does about what is happening during those long nights of tossing and turning. After all, who would worry about not getting enough sleep if they were getting enough?

The answer seems obvious: no one. But that is not necessarily the case. People who do not have to perform at their peak the next day, who do not have to spend long hours driving or doing tedious tasks at computers and on assembly lines, who do not have to make split-second decisions that could save or lose a life, who do not have to brainstorm in boardrooms under the scrutiny of their bosses, basically everyone who does not have to produce at top efficiency the next day, can live with less-than-enough sleep more easily. People who can nap the following afternoon, work according to their own rhythms, and even utilize the lack-of-sleep slowness to observe, reflect, and respond spaciously, do well enough. Insomnia undoubtedly has its miseries, but it is the demands we make upon ourselves by day that turn those miseries into nightmares.

In the industrialized West, people have been worrying about not getting enough sleep for more than a century, even when they were getting more than we do now. Our twenty-first-century concern with sleep, and the lack of it, is nothing new. Nor is the blaming of modern life, the proliferation of advice, or the platitudes about living with less stress. The word *insomnia* entered the English language in the 1700s, and it appears that the condition itself did not become prevalent, or a matter of public concern, until the end of the nineteenth century, when industrialization was in full swing. Professor Jim Horne, who runs the Sleep Research Centre at Loughborough University, unearthed a remarkable editorial from the September 29, 1894, issue of the *British Medical Journal* that addressed the issue:

> The subject of sleeplessness is once more under public discussion. The hurry and excitement of modern life is held to be responsible for much of the insomnia of which we hear; and most of the articles and letters are full of good

> advice to live more quietly and of platitudes concerning the harmfulness of rush and worry.[29]

Adults have also been concerned about the amount of sleep their children get for a long time. In 2012, researchers at the University of South Australia published a comprehensive review of studies of children's sleep from 1897 through 2009, revealing that experts have always wanted children to sleep longer than they were.[30] However, the number of hours recommended have slowly declined (by a total of seventy-five minutes) over the past century, and the amount of sleep kids actually got decreased at the same pace. In the early parts of the twentieth century, electric lights and radio were blamed for stealing children's sleep; today it is social media and video games. Tim Olds, who worked on the study, added: "Throughout the 100-hundred year period, we have been blaming whatever the new technology is—radio, TV, the internet."

The relatively new field of sleep medicine has many recommendations for improving the ability to fall and stay asleep: get exercise and exposure to natural light during the day, eat well, quiet down in the evening, avoid alcohol and caffeine, create a safe dark place to sleep, put aside worries, computers and smartphones, go to bed and wake up at the same times every day, and so on. If problems continue, a sleep study is in order to rule out apnea, a breathing disorder that affects many children and adults who have no idea why they have so much difficulty managing their days. Experts also recommend a short course of cognitive-behavioral therapy to develop good sleep practices and attitudes. Sleeping pills are considered by most to be a last resort. Even so, the CDC revealed in 2009 that 11 percent of adults interviewed reported that they *never* got enough rest or sleep during the previous thirty days.[31]

Chronic, unremitting insomnia usually cannot be attributed to a particular reason or condition. The newborn babies, broken hearts, busy brains, physical injuries, young loves, and sudden losses that can sabotage sleep for most of us at times are not the primary issues for confirmed insomniacs. Even when their lives are going well and they do all the recommended things to ensure sleep, it does not happen more than a few hours a night. The switch simply will not flip. Exhaustion settles in. Minds never clear, and emotions run raw. Living life at wit's end requires insomniacs to employ all the self-discipline they can muster—and more—to shuffle through their days and nights. Remarkably, many manage to achieve great things despite the toll that sleeplessness takes on their health, careers, and relationships. I have a good friend who managed to work for years as a criminal defense attorney on a few hours' sleep a night, but the struggle just about killed her.

Worry about sleep has become something of a habit in the West during the last few centuries, one that has spread throughout the world in recent years with the expansion of the global economy. It is both symbol and symptom of the stresses of contemporary life, whatever the age and circumstances. Even though the causes of insomnia are usually located in larger socioeconomic contexts, be it the hectic pace of modern living, the prevalence of shift work, or new-fangled technology, the solutions offered are inevitably individual. Experts address the sleepers, rather than their employers or the city light department, with their lists of things to do and not do. If their suggestions were truly effective, though, insomnia would not be the problem it is today. When sleep continues to evade us, fault is often found in the (non)sleeper's state of mind or lack of compliance. As the editorial from the *British Medical Journal* concluded, "The pity is that so many people are unable to follow the good advice and are obliged to lead a life of anxiety and high tension."[32]

We want to believe that it is within our powers to sleep, or not sleep, when it often is not, as any insomniac, narcoleptic, or sleepwalker will tell you, and much to the delight of the makers of our endless supply of sleeping potions and energy drinks. It is a peculiarly modern Western notion, this idea that we can, and should, control our bodies. Sleep defies that illusion, for it is fundamentally a physiological process orchestrated by a fluctuating body chemistry that goes about its business without our conscious involvement, and often in spite of our wishes.

Sleep Fragility

After all of the theories have been explored, one fact remains: sleep is fragile. All manner of conditions (heat, cold, good food, bad food, solitude, company, noise, silence, love and the loss of love, and so on) can fray its fabric, and there is little we can do to reliably improve it, as chronic insomniacs remind us. The fabric of sleep requires trust and a sense of safety to remain intact, and these qualities come by way of grace, good genes, viable relationships, and practice, more than anything else.

The fast-paced life of anxiety and high tension many encounter in postindustrial cultures further erodes that fabric. Societies may undergo enormous social, economic, and political changes, totally transforming the lives of their members, but they leave it up to individuals to successfully adapt, stay calm, and keep sleeping. Our sleep, by virtue of its vulnerability and uncontrollability, displays the strain of our efforts to accommodate to that which is not always suited to us, be it work demands or LED screens, long before we realize the stretch may be too great. There are simple things societies can do, such as delaying school start times for adolescents, providing flexible work schedules for adults, changing the color of light that electronics emit, and building workplaces with windows and skylights to expose employees to daylight to improve both sleep and daytime alertness, but the political will is often lacking.[33]

I also suspect that modern Americans, who most likely learned to sleep alone in quiet darkness as infants, are less equipped neurologically to shift into and out of waking and sleeping states. After all, as anthropologist Carol Worthman observed with befuddled curiosity, we put our infants to sleep in silent, dark rooms under minimal sensory loads, "but later expect [them] to titrate arousal and focus attention appropriately in a world with high sensory loads and heavy competing demands for attention."[34] Intriguingly, foreign-born Americans are more likely to sleep the recommended six to eight hours a night than their native-born counterparts.[35] While the reasons for this disparity are unknown, it cannot be because immigrants work less or experience less stress; the opposite is more likely to be true. Could it be that most immigrants were raised in cultures that provide infants more of a continuum of care when their nervous systems are developing, enabling them to handle stress and sleep more easily?

If learning to sleep as an infant meant crying it out alone, it would be easy to imagine that a physiological condition of hyperarousal could become the norm, making it difficult to calm down and relax, keeping restful sleep at bay for years to come. Some of us may be wired that way from the start (as parents of colicky babies suspect), while others become so over time as a result of trauma, ongoing stress, or simply by aging and losing the deep, SW sleep that sustains our capacities to calm down.

Primary insomnia (that is not a symptom or side effect of something else) is increasingly considered to be a function of autonomic hyperarousal, usually indicated by some combination of elevated body temperature and heart rate, increased high-frequency brain wave activation, higher levels of cortisol and adrenaline, and decreased levels of melatonin.[36] In short, wakeful vigilance routinely overcomes relaxed sleepiness by night—and by day. We are too awake, rather than not sleepy enough. The result, combined with a genetic propensity toward anxiety, makes for a chronic insomniac. While most of us who struggle with sleep fall short of that label, I suspect the same physiological forces, emotional states, and socioeconomic conditions tug at our hold of sleep.

Fortunately, our nervous systems continue to grow and learn, building new connections, discarding old ones, and facilitating shifts in hormonal balances. Just as we can learn how to play bridge, lift weights, or do the two-step, we can train ourselves to shift into and out of states of mind, body, and emotion, even to shut off the default mode network that keeps our minds busy. We can cultivate our abilities to calm down, let go, go within, and drift off, to counteract the tendencies to gear up, grab on, look out, and get ahead that are so encouraged in our society.

There are a variety of tools available to help us downshift; meditation, yoga, and biofeedback (including neurofeedback) have all been shown to be effective in improving sleep.[37] They are not quick or easy, though, and what works for one person may not help the next. But they can be well worth trying before opening the medicine cabinet and reaching for that bottle of sleeping pills.

7

DOWNERS, BENZOS, AND Z-DRUGS: THE COMMERCIALIZATION OF SLEEP

As much as I tried to explain to my seven-year-old stepdaughter why we needed to lie down for hours every night, her fury at this artificially imposed limitation to her days never abated. As a parent, I had expected to have to justify other cruelties of life, like getting vaccinations or being called names, but I never imagined that I would have to defend sleep. After all, I considered it to be one of life's greatest blessings. But Lauren was a night owl, and she struggled to fit into the strict schedules of her school and our work. She was rarely tired when it came time to go to bed, often lay awake for hours at night, and usually had to be strenuously coaxed out of bed, groggy and grumpy, in the morning. To this day, she remains the same.

We employed a variety of remedies to steer Lauren toward sleep in the evenings. We gave her a bedtime snack of warm milk and toast, played soothing music, and read stories in bed. When she was afraid of monsters, we strung imaginary rainbows between all the corners of her room to protect her. But the most successful of all our efforts was a mantra we made up and recited repeatedly before parting: "I will wake rested, refreshed, and ready for the day. I will wake rested, refreshed, and ready for the day…" I still use that formula for restorative sleep when I know I'll need it.

Lauren had an easier time with sleep on the weekends, and we assumed it was because our schedules were more relaxed outside the demands of school and work. She stayed up later and slept in longer, which made all of us much happier. Then, upon learning that Lauren was trading her healthy, homemade lunches for chocolate cake at school and was drinking Dr Peppers at a friend's house on the way home, we realized that sugar and caffeine were probably interfering with her sleep during the week. They may have even contributed to her bedtime fear of monsters, which she did not develop until second grade. Much as we tried, there was no way we could keep Lauren from the chemical carousal of modern life.

It would be trouble enough if that chemical carousal were limited to caffeinated drinks, sugary foods, or nightcaps, but it is not. My grandmother, who woke at three every morning and could not fall back asleep, decided to learn how to type Braille. She rented a machine and tapped away every morning until the sun rose. Today, she would have probably been diagnosed with terminal insomnia and given a prescription for one of many available sleep medications. That is what happened to an 82-year-old friend of mine, whose insomnia was treated with a popular benzodiazepine. It seemed to help her sleep a little longer, but she began falling in the mornings—a dangerous thing for a woman her age. When she met with her doctor about it, he gave her a stimulant to take every morning to wake up more fully. She wanted to stop taking her sleep medication, but the broken bones and bruises from her falls made sleep even more difficult. Like many others, my friend is caught in the sedation-stimulation loop, the dizzying spin of the chemical carousal.

A History of Sleep Aids

Historical records suggest that sleep has never been easy. There have always been dangers afoot in the dark and reasons for a multitude of anxieties to arise when we close our eyes, not to mention the ordinary noises, flickering lights, pesky insects, and pangs of love and hunger and that keep many awake today. Throughout most of history, people slept in groups and woke frequently to tend to fires, babies, and animals or to keep watch while the others slept. By the time writing was invented, the Greeks and Egyptians had already learned to extract opium from poppies to facilitate sleep. They also used mandrake root with wine to relieve pain, valerian root to calm the nerves, chamomile flowers and henbane seeds to ease the slide into slumber.

Good sleep, as we have come to call it, has rarely been assumed or expected. It was a favor bestowed by the gods, a reward for right living, a privilege of wealth, or the gift of darkness throughout the ages. People sought peaceful sleep the way hunters pursued prey and gatherers searched for nuts and roots to carry them through lean times. Sleep was like food, a cherished and necessary—though not always available—source of physical and spiritual sustenance.

The first chemically synthesized sleep medications were developed in nineteenth-century Europe. The most popular, chloral hydrate, depressed the central nervous system so much, it came to be used as a knock-out drug. It was made famous by Michael "Mickey" Finn, a bartender in Chicago who slipped it into the drinks of unsuspecting patrons to lift the money from their pockets, giving rise to the phrase *slipping a Mickey*.[1] Bromide, developed for its ability to calm seizures, was more prevalent in the later part of the nineteenth century. A British physician working in Shanghai, Dr. Neil Macleod, created a big stir in the medical field when he induced lengthy sleep with high doses of bromide to cure a patient's morphine addiction. *Merck's Archives* of 1897 described the treatment:

> For from five to nine days the patient sleeps incessantly and cannot be aroused, cannot walk, stand, sit, speak, or carry on any of the higher cerebral functions... Following this sleep is a gradual recovery of the powers of locomotion, speech, thought, etc., the progress being daily visible, lasting about a fortnight.[2]

Bromide was one of the first drugs to be used successfully to alleviate a major psychiatric illness, and the discovery proved to be a great boon for the nascent psychopharmaceutical industry. In fact, the story of the succession of sleep medications developed over the last two centuries is emblematic of the promise and perils of psychopharmacology in general.

In the early twentieth century, barbiturate compounds replaced chloral hydrate and bromide as the drugs of choice for sleep. Downers, as they were commonly called, were prescribed for seizures, anxiety, pain, and insomnia. On the street, they came to be known as barbies, goofballs, red devils, bumble bees, bluebirds, pink ladies, and dolls (as popularized in the 1967 film *Valley of the Dolls*). Production in the United States increased more than 400 percent during the Great Depression and continued to boom during World War II, when soldiers serving in the South Pacific were given goofballs to help them tolerate the extreme heat and prevent "combat anxiety," a clinical term for the fear of being killed.

Back home, pharmaceutical companies that relied on prescription drugs like penicillin were beginning to lose money, and the future of the industry looked grim. In response, as historian

Andrea Tone described in *The Age of Anxiety*, company executives decided to develop their own patent-protected, high-price drugs to treat common ailments associated with cardiovascular disorders, degenerative diseases, and mental problems.[3] Drugs of the mind, as they were called at the time, proved to be their cash cows. In 1954, a tranquilizer called Miltown (after the town where it was manufactured) hit the market, and it soon became the first psychotropic blockbuster in history. Miltown, sometime called the peace pill and emotional aspirin, successfully medicalized common anxieties that appeared to be increasing as men and women sought to fit themselves into a booming postwar economy and gendered social structure that valued productivity, efficiency, and stability above all else.

Barbiturates like Miltown were widely advertised, promoted to physicians by hordes of drug company representatives known as detail men, and readily prescribed to people for a host of emotional problems, from the "executive stomach" to the "housewives' nerves." By 1955, the United States manufactured enough barbiturates annually to treat ten million people, despite increasing evidence that they were highly addictive and potentially lethal, especially in combination with alcohol.[4]

One of the most notorious barbiturates, thalidomide, was sold worldwide as a sleep aid and cure for morning sickness from 1957 until it was found to be the cause of birth defects in more than eight thousand babies a few years later.[5] Considered one of the worst tragedies in pharmaceutical history, the thalidomide disaster prompted countries worldwide to strengthen regulatory control over medications made available to the general public. In the United States, Congress passed a law requiring manufacturers to demonstrate the safety and efficacy of new drugs and to obtain approval from the Food and Drug Administration (FDA) before distribution.

In 1962, President Kennedy, who regularly took a slew of drugs, including Ritalin for energy, barbiturates for sleep, codeine for pain, and Librium for anxiety, established a special committee to investigate drug dependence.[6] At the time, an estimated two hundred fifty thousand Americans were addicted to barbiturates, including Marilyn Monroe, who died from an overdose that year. The use and abuse of barbiturates did not decline until the 1970s, when the FDA started regulating sleep medications as controlled substances and when safer sedatives, known as benzodiazepines, were introduced.

Most people recognize the names under which benzos were (and are) sold—Valium, Xanax, Klonopin, Ativan, and others. Although hypnosis and mental relaxation had already been proven effective treatments for insomnia by the time these drugs hit the market, benzodiazepines were quick and easy—reducing anxiety, relaxing muscles, and inducing sleep at the first pop of the chill pill. Benzodiazepines are not recommended for use longer than two to four weeks, primarily because of the risk of dependence. However, many physicians continue to prescribe them once emergencies have passed, often at the requests of their patients who are unable to tolerate withdrawal.[7] Withdrawal from benzodiazepines can be wicked, usually causing prolonged agitation and worsened insomnia, a fact that most first-time users do not realize, and these symptoms can last for months, even years.[8] Short-term use can lead consumers, unwittingly, into a lifetime of dependence and gradual deterioration of physical and mental health. Anne Milton, the public health minister in the United Kingdom, told the BBC in 2011: "I've met people who've been addicted to some of these drugs for twenty or thirty years—wrecked their lives, wrecked their jobs, wrecked their families. It's a silent addiction."[9] I have friends who cannot get more than a few hours of sleep without their prescribed benzos, and they endure the side effects of morning drowsiness, dizziness, and memory loss on a daily basis because the rebound insomnia is so much worse.

As the risks of taking prescription sleep aids became more known, people turned to over-the-counter antihistamine drugs. The FDA in the US began regulating these products in the late 1970s, approving antihistamines as hypnotics for transient insomnia. When used occasionally, many find them effective; however, it is easy to develop tolerance with regular use, and they rarely impact entrenched, chronic insomnia. Herbal and hormonal sleep aids, which often include valerian or melatonin, are not regulated by the FDA and are often discouraged by medical professionals; however, they work well for many, especially shift workers needing to change their sleep-wake schedules. Surveys indicate that approximately 10 percent of the general population uses over-the-counter sleep medications.[10]

The next generation of powerful hypnotic sleeping pills, known as nonbenzodiazepines, were developed, tested, approved, and offered for public consumption in the 1990s. Sold as Ambien (Zolpidem), Sonata (Zalepon), and Lunesta (Eszopiclone), they are shorter acting and less addictive, and they usually do not result in a hangover the next day. Even so, withdrawal can be difficult if used nightly for more than a few weeks. The nonbenzodiazepines, often known as Z-drugs, have become immensely popular. When Colin Powell was the US secretary of state with a punishing schedule of oversees travels, he told a prominent Arab journalist: "Everybody uses Ambien."[11] He was not exaggerating much. In 2005, more than twenty-six million prescriptions for Ambien were written in the United States, totaling more than $2 billion.[12] In the UK, half a million prescriptions for the drug are handed out each year.[13]

People have been known to talk, walk, shop, cook, text, binge eat, have sex, and drive while asleep on Ambien, with no memory of doing so afterward. A nurse in Denver took Ambien before bed and rose a few hours later, got in her car, began driving, caused an accident, urinated in the middle of an intersection, and became violent with police officers—without ever waking up.[14] In St. Louis, a security systems representative returned from a sales trip, ate pork chops and salad for dinner, took an Ambien, and went to bed. When police arrested her hours later, she had no memory of starting a bath, leaving the water running, jumping into her Mini Cooper with her dog, running a red light on her way to a local diner, and crashing into a car.[15] Even though episodes like these are rare, an ongoing survey of US toxicology labs is revealing that Ambien alone often makes it into the top-ten list of drugs found in impaired drivers,[16] and visits to the ER linked to the nonbenzodiazepines increased a whopping 220 percent between 2005 and 2010.[16] Z-drugs are so commonly used, the phenomenon has prompted portrayals of Ambien zombies and has even provided the basis for criminal defense in court.[18]

In 2007, the FDA responded by requiring manufactures of Ambien, Lunesta, and eleven other brands of sleeping pills to warn consumers of "possible adverse events." The warnings have not dampened sales any more than those on cigarette packages did. The following year (when actor Heath Ledger died of an accidental overdose of prescription drugs, including sleeping pills), American pharmacists filled more than fifty-six million prescriptions for sleep medications, a 70 percent increase from 2002.[19] This dramatic increase, especially among teens, has been attributed to the FDA's 1997 decision to allow drug companies to advertise directly to consumers.[20]

Since then, it has been hard to watch a television program in the US without seeing Lunesta's luna moth fluttering around the bed of a sound sleeper, hearing Ambien's midnight rooster crow, or being told by Rozerem that our dreams miss us. As drug companies compete through advertising, sales have risen accordingly. In 2004, a healthcare consumer advocacy organization gave its Bitter Pill Award to the manufacturers of Ambien and Lunesta for "overmarketing insomnia medications to anyone who's ever had a bad night's sleep."[21]

The Sleep Industry

Today, sleeping pills are among the most advertised, most prescribed, and most profitable drugs in the world, even though their effectiveness has been shown to be minimal at best.

That's right. An analysis of sleeping pill studies conducted by the National Institutes of Health and published in 2007 revealed that sleep medications, including the nonbenzodiazepines, reduce the time it takes to fall asleep by an average of 12.8 minutes compared with placebos and increase the total sleep time by only 11.4 minutes. Moreover, functioning does not improve the next day.[22]

I can hear my friends who take Ambien nightly protest that it is not true, insisting they sleep more and do better the next day with the drug. However, lab studies consistently report that people think they get more sleep when they take medication than they actually do.[23] Sleep researcher Allan Rechtschaffen once invited a group of people who described themselves as good sleepers and another group who saw themselves as poor sleepers into his lab for the night. When they had been asleep for ten minutes (judging by their behavior and brain wave patterns), Rechtschaffen woke them and asked them what they had been doing. The good sleepers claimed to be sleeping, while the poor sleepers insisted they had been awake the entire time. After confirming the results in further experiments, Rechtschaffen tried giving the self-described insomniacs a sleeping pill one night and a placebo the next. Remarkably, they insisted they had been sleeping on the night with the pill and had remained awake the night with the placebo. The results were the same for Halcion, a benzodiazepine, and for Ambien, a nonbenzodiazepine. It appears that the sleeping pills did more to change the subjects' perception of waking and sleeping than it changed the brain waves themselves.

This effect is nothing to sneeze at. It is a wonderful trick—and a mystery that confounds many researchers. Some propose that sleep medications work primarily by reducing anxiety, leaving us feeling more rested and carefree come morning. Others suggest that the retrograde amnesia induced by sedative-hypnotic medications erases our memories of tossing and turning, leaving us with the notion that we have been "out" all night. Regardless of the cause, the impression of refreshing sleep is a relief in itself because it chips away at the vicious cycle of anxiety and insomnia that wears many down to despair.

Sleep scientists have shown for some time that insomniacs think they sleep less than they do. Sleep expert Stanley Coren tells a great story to illustrate the point.[24] He opened his eyes one morning believing that he had not slept a wink all night, ready to complain about it to his wife, when he noticed white powder and chunks of plaster on top of the bed. Looking up, he saw that parts of the ceiling had cracked and fallen during the night. Then he turned on the news and learned he had slept through a major earthquake, the one that struck the San Francisco Bay Area during the World Series in 1989.

If we are so capable of misperceiving the amount of sleep we lose, it makes sense that we could do the same with the amount we get. Anxiety about sleep not only adds to the misery of sleeplessness; it also fuels the perception that we are not sleeping even when we are. Isn't that the nature of anxiety, to worry about something that is not happening but could occur at some future time? The fact that sleep medications can offer the impression of refreshing sleep in its absence is immensely helpful.

However, sleep medications do not restore healthy sleep cycles; they simply hide and intercept disordered ones, perpetuating the problem—and the need for intervention.[25] The primary advantage they offer is a reduction in the time it takes to fall asleep, leaving us with less room to worry and drum up the anxieties that ward off sleep. They do not facilitate restorative deep sleep, nor do they address the factors that create and maintain insomnia. To get at the root of our problems with sleep, sleep medicine professionals claim we need to make changes in the ways we live, sleep, and even think.

That may seem like a tall order, but experts have adapted a short-term educational therapy called cognitive behavioral therapy (CBT) to do just that. CBT teaches people good waking and sleeping habits (the behavioral part) and shows them how to change their thinking to reduce anxiety (the cognitive part).[26] Clients learn the essentials of sleep hygiene (a term that epitomizes the medicalization of sleep, in my mind), including the importance of exercise and exposure to natural light during the day, winding down and avoiding chemical and electronic stimulants before bed, and creating a dark and peaceful place to sleep. They are encouraged to avoid napping and to reduce the time they spend in bed to a bare minimum so that when they finally lie down, the pressure to sleep is irresistible. Therapists also teach stress management techniques, such as progressive muscle relaxation, self-hypnosis, meditation, and putting aside worries to calm the body and mind. This last technique reminds me of the way Napoleon Bonaparte prepared for bed: "Different subjects… are arranged in my head as in a cupboard. When I wish to interrupt one train of thought, I shut that drawer and open another. Do I wish to sleep, I simply close all the drawers."

The most interesting part of CBT for insomnia, to my mind, is the cognitive component, in which therapists address the anxieties that beset the sleepless by "changing faulty beliefs and misconceptions about sleep."[27] They tell their clients that they may actually be getting more sleep than they believe (because people often think they are awake when, in fact, they are experiencing light sleep) and probably do not need as much sleep as they think. Most people, some add, need only five and a half hours of core sleep to maintain alertness the next day.

Sleep medicine professionals sometimes seem to be talking out of both sides of their mouths. On the one hand, we are told that even modest sleep restriction, from six to eight hours, is associated with daytime sleepiness and performance decline;[28] on the other hand, we are told not to worry, that it turns out we do not need all that sleep after all. It is all in our heads. Regardless, CBT has been shown to be as effective—if not more so—than medication in the treatment of insomnia in numerous studies, and the gains seem to last well.[29] CBT is a way of taking back one's sleep—and one's life. But it requires time and effort, something that many people feel they cannot afford, and it is often unavailable, so medication sales continue to rise.

While the world economy sputters and falters, the sleep industry is booming. Sleep aids are, as one article put it, a "bright spot in a sluggish economy."[30] Prescription and over-the-counter medications, sleep studies, white noise machines, earplugs, eye masks, apnea devices, sleep monitors, specialty mattresses, high-thread-count sheets, aromatherapy pillows, high-end beds, and alarm clocks fuel a sleep economy worth more than $20 billion a year in the US, and it is growing at a rate of 20 percent a year. It has been said that "sleep is the new sex," with Ambien filling in for Viagra since it became available generically.[31]

Sleep Anxiety

How did sleeping pills become so popular, despite their limited effectiveness and potentially dangerous side effects? It could be considered a perfect storm of factors: the increasing demands for work time and productivity in a teetering economy, round-the-clock commerce and media access, reduced amounts and quality of sleep, greater understanding of the dangers and long-term effects of sleep loss, and the medicalization of sleep with its plethora of diagnoses and treatments, all against the background of a culture that relies on stimulants to foster speed, productivity, and efficiency.

Employees often work overtime and outside their job descriptions for fear of losing their jobs if they refuse. Cutbacks and downsizing have further increased workloads, making it all the more necessary to operate at the top of one's game all day long, without any lapses. Fear of what one night of lost sleep could do to one's appearance and performance the next day has become a common concern.

However, even when people worked more than fifty hours a week under deplorable conditions at the beginning of the twentieth century, they still slept a good nine hours a night, so there must be more involved.[32] The nights were dark back then, for one thing. Electric lights did not reach most Western homes until the 1930s. By the end of the decade, radio was woven into the fabric of life, and television followed suit in the next two decades. When I was a child growing up in the 1950s and 1960s, television and radio went off the air at midnight; now, they never stop broadcasting. Computers, internet banking, and all-night convenience stores keep us plugged in to the news, business trends, and advertisements of the global economy all day and all night.

We now average six and a half hours of sleep a night, according to surveys conducted by the National Sleep Foundation (NSF), a 20 percent decrease in the last one hundred years, and one and a half hours less than in 1960.[33]

The NSF was founded in 1990 when a consortium of sleep doctors and researchers, known as the American Sleep Disorders Association, sought to educate the public about the importance of sleep.[34] It launched its first public education campaign in 1991 with the release of a sleep problems survey funded by the Searle drug company, which was seeking approval for the sale of its blockbuster new sleeping pill, Ambien (Zolpidem), at the time. That first year, the foundation also provided tutorials to primary care physicians on the diagnosis and treatment of sleep disorders, responded to more than eighteen thousand requests for information, and initiated a public information campaign on the problem of drowsy driving.

Since then, the NSF has published annual sleep surveys, informing the public of some stunning facts about sleep: 20 percent of those surveyed reported sleeping less than six hours a night. Approximately one-third had fallen asleep at the wheel during the previous year, accounting for more than one hundred thousand accidents per year, and nearly one-third have nodded off at work during the past month, resulting in more than $18 billion dollars in lost productivity.[35]

While the NSF has been outlining the extent, costs, and dangers of sleep loss during the past twenty years, the new field of sleep medicine has been revealing the toll it takes on our health. Researchers have linked insufficient sleep to obesity, diabetes, heart disease, anxiety, depression, substance abuse, and immune suppression.[36] They have also demonstrated that inadequate sleep reduces our ability to pay attention, react in a timely manner, and make sound judgments, while triggering irritability and impulsivity, all of which increase the risk of serious accidents. In less than twenty years, sleep medicine professionals have defined how much sleep we need to function well, identified the signs of inadequate sleep, turned a private affair into public matter, transformed variations from the norm into pathologies, and named more than eighty sleep disorders, leading to the establishment of thousands of centers to diagnose and treat those disorders. The field of sleep medicine continues to grow as well; over five thousand sleep scientists from around the world attended the 27th Annual Meeting of Associated Professional Sleep Societies in 2013.

This medicalization of sleep and its disorders has enabled millions to access everything from sleeping pills to sleep studies and CPAP machines, for which many are immensely grateful.[37] It has also provided an enormous boon for pharmaceutical companies, sleep device manufacturers, researchers, and service providers. NHS spending on sleeping pills rose from £42 million in 2007 to £49.2 million in 2011—an increase of more than 17 percent.[38] In the popular consciousness, sleep has joined the ranks of diet and exercise as an essential for good health. Conversely, we have added insomnia to cigarettes and cholesterol on that growing list of things that can kill us.

Now that two-thirds of Americans report that they do not get enough sleep during weeknights, and they have learned that drowsy driving is comparable to driving drunk, sleepy eating expands the waistline and shortens the lifespan, and working tired is sloppy and inefficient, the fear of not getting enough is palpable. No wonder one in four Americans is willing to take a sleep aid at least once a year to rest assured that they are getting enough sleep.[39]

The ancient Greeks named a slew of troubles that were born of their goddess of the night, Nyx. They included blame, doom, retribution, deceit, strife, misery, and fate; in short, those worries, regrets, and resentments that proliferate endlessly under the cover of darkness, keeping us awake, wide-eyed, and worked up in the night-world of Nyx. Modern sleep aids quiet that restless brood, for better or for worse. However, they rarely remain quiet for long. Nyx was also the mother of the day goddess, Hemera, and her restless brood has a way of slipping into our day lives when we are not looking. Dawn and dusk, those quivering junctures between Night and her daughter Day, often give shelter to our troubles, but the phantoms that populate our dreams drift into our waking lives more than we would like to think.

The very fact that we, as human beings, inhabit dreaming and waking worlds has intrigued, confounded, and frightened people the world over. Much as we may try to draw a clear line between our waking and dreaming lives to establish some semblance of order and control, nothing can keep the two from mingling.

8

THE SOCIAL DIVIDE: SEPARATING SLEEP FROM CONSCIOUSNESS

When I was nine or ten, I got a long sliver in the palm of my hand from running it along a weather-beaten wooden railing. My mother pulled out the exposed end with tweezers, but the rest festered in my hand for days. When red streaks appeared one morning, she took me downtown to the family physician. I remember sitting on the end of the table in the small examination room, swinging my legs furiously while the doctor placed the blade of a scalpel against my skin, made a small incision, and pulled the skin apart, and I fainted.

At the time, I did not know what had happened. My memory is of being laid out under the bright lights of an operating room while a doctor in a white coat and green mask patiently worked on me for hours with a nurse assisting from the other side. When I woke up to a little bottle of smelling salts pressed under my nostrils, the family doctor told me I had fainted for a second. I objected, insisting that I had had an operation in another room, but he glanced at my mother with that isn't-she-precious look and asked how I was doing.

I never knew what to call that experience. Was it a dream, a hallucination, or a paradoxically unconscious awareness of what was happening? Nor have I been able to understand what state I was in for those few seconds. Was I momentarily asleep, temporarily unconscious, or translated into another world? These are the questions people have asked about experiences in sleep for millennia.

Syncope

There is a medical term for what happened to me: syncope. Defined as a transient loss of consciousness, the word also refers to contractions that omit one or more sounds from a word and to rhythms that skip a beat or stress a weak one. The meanings focus upon what is missing from the overriding pattern. They define what happens in the terms of absence, rather than presence, excluding, by definition, all the wild and woolly things that can occur in the span of a missing beat. My syncope on the doctor's table shares two key qualities with sleep: the solitariness of having encounters that are not shared—or even recognized—by others and an uncanny, out-of-the-ordinary sense of time.

Time is a slippery thing, an abstract concept that we cannot see, hear, taste, or feel with our ordinary senses. Despite our commonsense notion that time is universal, Einstein demonstrated that it is relative to the individual observer and strangely elastic. Our brains actually construct our perception of time to put events in sequence, and the importance of those events may determine how long or short a passage of time seems to us. We feel time slow in the face of danger, stand still at historic moments, and fly by when we are actively engaged. Hours collapse into what feels like an instant when we are soundly asleep. On the other hand, dreams can unfold epic tales within the span of a five-minute nap. Past and future events occasionally appear in the present moment. Time is so subjective, we need clocks to keep us in step with a shared, standardized sense of a day's (and a night's) progression.

The mercurial quality of time in sleep has prompted some cultures, such as those of ancient Greek, East Indian, and Tibetan peoples, to define two separate coexisting times correlating with different modes of perception.[1] There is the ordinary sense of time we share with others and experience as the passage of events with a distinct past, present, and future, and another extraordinary perception of a sacred time in which all that has been and will be is folded into the present moment. In Tibetan Buddhism, this sacred time is only knowable in the clear light of ultimate reality.

According to the Dalai Lama, we can catch a glimpse of clear light reality when we sneeze, faint, die, have sex, or fall fast asleep—when our normally "strong sense of self is slightly relaxed."[2] From this perspective, the extraordinary experiences that occasionally come upon us when we slip from one state of consciousness into another may not be distorted impressions or absences of awareness at all. They may be clear, momentarily unclouded glimpses of a greater reality beyond the familiar one we inhabit by day.

These syncopes, or eclipses of ordinary awareness, break the continuity of shared time and place, catapulting us into uniquely individual worlds that expire the moment we come back to reality as we know it. It is like a cutaway in a movie, when (before the digital age) a filmstrip was sliced and taped to a strip from a different scene so viewers switched instantly from one place and time to another. A similar shift occurs every time we slip into and out of sleep and the dream worlds within.

Negotiating the Divide

Sometimes, especially when I wake from a strong dream or a deep sleep, it takes me a little while to figure out where I am, what day it is, and what I have to do next. It is as if my day world puts itself back together piece by piece. From the standpoint of my sleeping self, I find this process of reconstituting my previous life an extraordinary marvel as I return to the exact place where I left off. My waking self, on the other hand, sees nothing remarkable in my daily resumption of reality and readily dismisses my nighttime adventures in order to pick up a new day.

As a child, the English novelist Gerald Bullett wondered how these worlds fit together and concluded that we must live double lives, one in each world. He explained:

> Sleeping and waking I supposed to be not two processes but two aspects of the same process. To fall asleep "here" is to wake "there." My head sinks gratefully into the pillow, and the world dissolves; and at that very moment, on another plane or planet, I rub my waking eyes and begin a new day, resuming without thought or sense of strangeness.[3]

It is hard to reconcile sleeping and waking realities, and every culture has its methods of guiding its members in negotiating the divide. The Mayans of Central America have a saying that advises people to "walk with a foot in each world," refusing to privilege one over the other.[4] Ancient Chinese literature, especially the fourth-century Taoist text *Liezi*, regards sleeping and waking worlds as equal counterparts in a greater whole, akin to night and day, winter and summer, and yin and yang. Sleeping and waking are viewed as reversible, like other polarities.[5] The oldest Hindu

Upanishads, including the *Prashna Upanishad*, value sleep over waking life as closer and more akin to an ultimate reality. African traditions honor sleep as a time when one can commune with the dead and receive guidance.[6] "In fact," wrote Mircea Eliade, a Romanian scholar of world religions, "'Sleep' is ridiculed only in Europe, only certain European peoples consider it a symbol of laziness, of stupidity and intellectual sterility. In other cultures, sleep is regarded as a state of perfect meditation, of autonomy and creation."[7]

The *Liezi* also portrayed a wide variation in the balance between sleeping and waking priorities in analogies of geographical terms.[8] In the southwest corner, people sleep almost all the time, waking only once every five years, and they believe dreams are reality and reality is a dream. In the opposite northeast corner, the inhabitants are awake all the time, aggressive and competitive, and they do not believe in dreams. In the middle, there is a balance between time spent asleep and awake, and people are creative and abundant. They know that dreams are dreams and reality is reality.

Contemporary psychiatrist and dream researcher Ernest Hartmann makes a similar distinction between people with "thin boundaries," who are most likely to remember dreams and experience reality as fluid, and those with "thick boundaries," who rarely recall dreams and easily keep time and space well organized.[9] The vast majority of us, Hartmann adds, fall somewhere between thick and thin. Many contemporary cultures, especially those influenced by Western worldviews, lean toward thicker boundaries, dismissing dreaming and other subjective experiences in favor of waking ones. The scheduled lives many lead, with distinct times and places for particular activities, foster these thicker boundaries. Historically, Western thinkers have ignored, and even forbidden, momentary experiences of surrendering or losing oneself in a preference for rationality, control, and individuality.[10] Sleep has become an "inadmissible abyss," to use a phrase from that brilliant insomniac, Vladimir Nabokov.[11]

We do not usually sit down and tell our children that dreams are not real; rather, the message becomes clear in what we do—and do not—acknowledge. When my family doctor ignored my claim that I had had an operation in another room, he effectively taught me to dismiss my subjective experience in order to belong to the shared realm of what others saw and heard. In explaining that I had fainted for a couple of seconds, he named and defined what had happened to me from an outside perspective, which was helpful, but it left me alone with an experience that had no place in that world. It was one of many encounters with adults that functioned to induct me into a collective worldview that defined experiences as either real or not real, true or made up.

Another of these encounters occurred the day I found my tooth in my mother's bureau drawer—the one I had left under my pillow for the tooth fairy, which, according to Germanic tradition, comes in the night to gather the fallen teeth of children and replace them with coins. I felt confused and betrayed, as I depended on my parents to explain the world and could not fathom why they would lie to me about it. To this day, I wonder why parents attribute their actions to fictional characters like Santa Claus, the Easter bunny, or the tooth fairy only to turn around and insist that their children stop making up stories and tell the truth. Then I remind myself of what happened next.

When I got my mother to confess that she was the tooth fairy (and forget that I had rifled through her drawers), I joined the confederacy of those in the know and promised to keep the secret from my little brother. I instantly felt more grown up and later enjoyed clandestine smiles with my older sisters when my brother talked about the tooth fairy. It was a rite of passage of sorts, an initiation into the world of grown-ups, where tangible things ruled and the intangible shriveled up like the Wicked Witch of the West into a puddle of nothingness. If I did not already know, I learned then that dreams are like Easter bunnies, childish fantasies we all outgrow.

I did not come from a family that shared and pondered dreams, visions, or mystical experiences. We did not marvel over miracles or pray to God for guidance. Instead, we reasoned things out, debated politics, and gave each other enormous freedom. In many ways, my family was typical of the Anglo-Saxon Protestant culture that has dominated much of the rhetoric and traditions of the United States and the United Kingdom. Belonging to that privileged group made it easy for me to be successful in school and elsewhere, but it also instilled a distrust of subjectivity that shuttered my world for many years.

Having found my baby teeth, I was happy to enter the world of the "real" and took to reading history and science with a vengeance. I did projects on the solar system with hanging styrofoam balls for planets, on early humankind with drawings of Neanderthal skulls, and on the cradle of civilization with a papier-mâché map of the Tigris and Euphrates Valleys. I believed everything I read, and it never occurred to me that Pluto would lose its status as a planet one day or that Africa would be found to have been the origin of humankind. History and science were not cultural interpretations in my book; they were absolute truths.

Then, in tenth grade, my English teacher asked us to write a story. It may seem like a simple request, but I was flummoxed. I did not know how to make things up; I only knew how to read and find out things. In desperation the night before the paper was due, I wrote about a strange experience I had had a few weeks before, when I was sick with a fever and found myself hovering a few feet over my body. Since that was not long enough, I added a segment from a recent dream. When I handed in the paper, I thought to myself: *Well, at least I was able to make up something.* In my mind at that time, dreams, stories, and most private experiences were collected in the category of make-believe, something only the young, the foolish, and a few English teachers would accept.

The following week, my teacher returned the paper with a note that read: "See me after class." When everyone else had left the room, he handed me a well-worn paperback book, *The Sleeping Prophet*, about the self-claimed American psychic Edgar Cayce,[12] leaned over, and whispered: "Don't tell anyone I gave this to you." Is there any better way to engage an adolescent?

I read the entire book that night, astonished to learn there was someone who asked the big questions in life that are close to any adolescent's heart and received the answers in his sleep. He advised thousands of people, including the likes of Woodrow Wilson, Thomas Edison, and George Gershwin, with the information he supposedly garnered from the land of Nod. That night, my questionable experiences—the nighttime dreams, daytime reveries and fainting episodes—began to assume legitimacy. They seemed more real and worth considering, and I started keeping a dream diary. The partitions I had learned to erect between real and make-believe, awake and asleep, conscious and unconscious, began to waver with uncertainty.

A Brief History of the Divide

Anthropologist Barbara Tedlock, who has reviewed much of the literature about sleep from many of the world's cultures, maintains that this sharp division between waking and slumbering realities, and its corollary dismissal of private, subjective experiences, is not universal but a Western European construction.[13] The notion has so infused the modern worldview shared by many across the globe that we assume it is the nature of reality, not an idea that structures our perceptions.

Tedlock traces this division back to the ancient Greeks, especially Aristotle, who brushed off dreams as mental pictures that—like reflections in water—are not real objects. But the dismissal of the interior life did not end there. In the Middle Ages, Christian leaders denounced dreams and visions as the work of the devil. The Scientific Revolution, in turn, shifted attention to collectively observable phenomena, making it easier to ignore subjective experiences because they could not be shared, measured, and quantified. While sleep had intrigued physicians, philosophers, and artists in the ancient and medieval worlds as a place of mystery and revelation, its mystique fell into disgrace during the Enlightenment. The waking state became the standard of reality and normalcy in the West, and sleep experiences began to be viewed as hallucinatory delusions. Goya's famous etching *The Sleep of Reason Produces Monsters* vividly portrays the monsters considered to be unleashed by sleep in the absence of reason.

Industrialization functioned to separate the workday and the night into distinct times and spaces. It also prioritized productivity, further marginalizing the hours spent in bed. Like a geological rift in the continent of Western civilization, the divide between day and night, objective and subjective, conscious and unconscious, grew wider over time.

However, there has also been a long, covert mystery tradition in the West that values individual subjective experiences, especially those that can be had "behind closed eyes and lips," as the etymology of the word *mystery* makes clear. From the Eleusinian Mysteries of ancient Greece through the rites of Jewish Kabbalists and Christian mystics to the Native American Church today, people have practiced: fasting, sensory deprivation, ritual, contemplation, dream incubation, song, and prayer—often accompanied by the use of sacred herbs—in search of a wisdom that can only be found within. Even though we have come to associate these revelatory practices with religion, it has been clear to many throughout Western history that there is nothing mystical or contradictory in the idea that everything that happens to us—all that we sense, perceive, intuit, and dream—is real and useful.

These mystery traditions, and their experience of the interior life, have been largely erased from the Western canon. When I learned about Pythagoras in school as a child, I was taught his famous mathematical theorem but never told that he was better known as a philosopher who was quoted as saying: "Sleep, dream and ecstasy are the three doors opening upon the Beyond, whence come to us the science of the soul." Nor did I learn about Synesius of Cyrene, a fifth-century Greek bishop who wrote of sleep: "We ought to seek this branch of knowledge before all else; for it comes from us, is within us, and is the special possession of the soul." In Synesius's view, sleep provides access to an inner wisdom that is not available to us by day. "One should consult one's bed," he admonished, as one would consult the oracle at Delphi." Fortunately, my tenth-grade English teacher was willing to take the risk to offer me a glimpse of that branch of knowledge when he handed me the book about Edgar Cayce, even if he did have to swear me to secrecy. While I will never know for sure why he asked me not to tell anyone about his gift, I can only presume he thought my parents might disapprove.

As human beings, we inherit the capacity—and the necessity—to inhabit two worlds. Our sleeping and waking lives are so interwoven, they cannot be fully separated, as much as we may try to choose one over the other. As the eighteenth-century French essayist Michel de Montaigne, one of the founders of the school of skepticism, observed: "Those who have compared our life to a dream were perhaps more right than they thought... Sleeping we are awake, and waking asleep." In one short sentence, Montaigne not only challenged the cultural preference for waking over sleeping; he also questioned the very distinction we make between the two—and suggested they actually overlap.

9

WHEN SLEEPING BIRDS FLY: HALF AWAKE AND HALF ASLEEP

During my first year in college, I dreamed that I had forgotten my children on a park bench in Europe, and I woke up believing it was true. It was a terrible realization that left me nearly paralyzed with guilt. When I finally managed to get out of bed, I knew I would have to quit school immediately and fly to Europe to retrieve my kids. I could hardly breathe for fear of what might have happened to them in my absence and of how long it would take me to get there and take them back into my arms. Not only that, I would have to admit what I had done to my adviser and drop out.

I headed straight over to his office, where I found a line of students sitting on the floor against the hallway wall, waiting to see him. I sat down at the end and waited, all the while rushing over all the details of getting a flight, searching for the park, going to the police, giving them the names and ages of my kids…but I could not remember their names and ages for the life of me. That was when it dawned on me that I had been dreaming.

The Permeable Boundary

For survival purposes, we need to be able to distinguish between our experiences of the outer world and those of our inner life, and people around the world usually do so effortlessly. Making clear demarcations between times and places for waking and sleeping may serve to keep us properly oriented. However, people with thin boundaries, like many artists, for instance, naturally experience mixtures of waking and sleeping states at times. Even those with thicker boundaries, who are not temperamentally inclined to confuse the two, find that certain conditions, such as jet lag, insomnia, and narcolepsy, destabilize the lines between waking and sleeping states to such an extent that each infects the other.

Narcolepsy, a chronic, neurological disorder affecting an estimated three million people worldwide, is characterized by excessive daytime sleepiness, fragmented night sleep, and sudden, uncontrollable attacks of sleep and muscle weakness that are socially devastating and potentially life threatening. A funny joke or a strong emotion can trigger these attacks without any notice. A sixty-three-year-old teacher with narcolepsy explained: "I'd be taking a bite of pie and my head would crash onto my plate."[1] Narcoleptics are also more prone to experiencing sleep paralysis, hypnagogic hallucinations, and episodes of sleepwalking. Understandably, the repeated intermingling of waking and sleeping states can create confusion as to what is really happening. An acquaintance of mine with intermittent narcolepsy looks at her dog, Sammy, whenever she is wondering if she is hallucinating events; if Sammy is sleeping peacefully as if nothing were going on, she concludes she must be dreaming, even if she thought she was awake.

Narcolepsy is an extreme case, but insomniacs, who are much more numerous, often feel stretched between the worlds of waking and sleeping without ever fully entering either, as if banned from the extremes and bound to the gray zones between. Almost everyone has experienced episodes of mixed sleep and waking states at times, especially when they are young, sick, recovering from surgery, changing work shifts, taking certain medications or drugs, or in great emotional distress. It also occurs, often unbeknownst to us, when we are just plain tired.

In 2008, physiologist James M. Krueger and his colleagues at the University of Wisconsin made a remarkable discovery about what happens when we are tired: small, independent clusters of neurons become fatigued from use, they release additional ATP and switch into sleep mode while the rest of the brain remains awake.[2] Their finding implies, as Krueger notes, that sleep "is not a whole-brain phenomenon," and that transitions between waking and sleeping may be more gradual and complex than previously thought. Furthermore, they do not seem to be directed by a central command center, like the sleep switch, but derived from an accumulation of actions taken by cell assemblies across the brain.

Researchers have observed that when one bundle of brain cells goes offline, neighboring ones tend to follow.[3] However, they do not fall in lines like dominoes; they catch on independently of the others in what appears to be a more complex, dynamic process. The clusters shifting into sleep mode begin to synchronize with each other, like swarms of fireflies or schools of minnows, building momentum until the entire brain catches on, the switch flips, and we nod off. Sleep, Krueger and his colleagues propose, is an emergent property of resonating cell assemblies, like the beehive that evolves from the bustling of a collection of bees without any direction from above.

When I tried to explain this to a friend, she said it reminded her of popping popcorn. The analogy is more accurate than she knew, for researchers report that they cannot predict which cluster will shut down next, just as we popcorn lovers do not know which kernel will pop next. Even so, the process eventually reaches a critical mass, triggering a flip of the sleep switch. That is the moment when sleep overcomes us.

Neither Awake nor Asleep, but Both

Krueger's discovery that sleep can occur in parts of the brain when the rest is awake was supported by research conducted by neuroscientist Chiara Cirelli and Giulio Tononi at the University of Wisconsin–Madison.[4] They called the phenomenon localized sleep, and demonstrated that it impairs performance and judgment. Tononi commented that these localized sleep states, which increase in frequency and length of time the longer we stay awake, are "more insidious [than total sleep] because we can't tell it's happening." They can also lead to brief episodes of total sleep, known as microsleep, which can last anywhere from a fraction of a second up to thirty seconds. The discovery of these surreptitious sleep states, whether they manifest as localized sleep or split-second dozing, has begun to erode the sharp boundaries we have erected between waking and sleeping states..

Biologists report that many birds and sea mammals have the ability to sleep with only one hemisphere of the brain at a time, called unihemispheric sleep.[5] Whales, dolphins, and seals cannot afford to shut down consciousness altogether because they are conscious breathers; when it is time to rest, they float on the surface of the water like logs or paddle in circles, keeping one half of their brains awake while the other half sleeps. Then they roll over or switch directions to give the other side a rest. Migratory birds employ a variety of half-asleep, half-awake states in order to cover great distances quickly. Even more sedentary birds, like mallard ducks, can sleep one hemisphere at a time. Since they typically sleep in rows, the ducks at the ends of the lines keep one eye open to watch for predators. Periodically, these guards turn around and switch places so the other half of their brains and bodies can sleep.

The fact that the guards turn around or switch places suggests that the half of their brains connected to their open eye gets tired and needs to sleep. In 2011, researchers tested this hypothesis by measuring the brain waves of several homing pigeons while they stayed up late watching David Attenborough's *The Life of Birds* with one eye covered.[6] They found that the parts of their brains that processed the visual information from the open eye did indeed tire and fall into a deeper sleep than the parts connected to the covered eye.

We may be more like these animals than we imagine. Yval Nir and colleagues at the University of Wisconsin and UCLA simultaneously recorded brain wave activity in multiple brain regions of neurosurgical patients and discovered that separate parts go off-line (and back online) at different times throughout the night, reflecting what the researchers called piecemeal sleep.[7] The fact that these regions simultaneously exhibited different sleep intensities made it clear that our sleep is not a global, uniform state but an ever-shifting patchwork quilt that responds to the previous day's activities. Many insomniacs report feeling neither awake nor asleep but rather something, to quote Shakespeare's *King Lear*, "'tween asleep and wake" that has qualities of both.

It makes sense. Look at the things we do when we have been up for a long time or have not been getting enough sleep. Our heads bob in front of the television while we insist we are still watching.

We put the car keys in the freezer and leave the ice cream melting on the table, cannot remember what we just read, or lose our cell phone even though we're talking on it. We discover that we passed our exit twenty miles ago or reach for a few potato chips only to discover that we have already eaten the entire bag. Many of these all-too-common incidents involve automatic behaviors, things we do without thinking, conscious knowledge, or control. Others would simply call it being absentminded, and that may well be a good description of what happens: some part of our minds is absent. It is asleep.

Split-second dreams can also occur when we are tired. Neurologist Oliver Sacks tells of a time years ago when he was reading the autobiography of an eighteenth-century deaf man before bed and came upon a wonderful description of deaf people signing with each other on the streets of London in the 1770s. He made a note to include a reference to this description in his next book, but when he looked for it the next day, it was not there. He had dreamed it. I have had similar experiences when I am so sleepy that I am beginning to nod off while watching a late-night movie, for instance, or pulling an all-nighter watching over someone who is dying. They are like little snippets of films, scenes from another place or time that engage me for a second or two and then evaporate. These are the moments when, as Sacks put it, "the doors of sleep swing wide open," even though we think we are awake.[8]

Just as we are not fully conscious when we are awake, it is also evident that we are not fully unconscious when we are asleep. People must remain aware of the positions of their bodies; otherwise, they would turn over one too many times and fall out of bed. Some sleepers, especially children and adolescents, walk, talk, eat, and even text in their sleep with no memory of doing so later. Mothers wake to the first whimpers of their babies, while the rest of the household remains asleep—an example of caretakers monitoring an environment unconsciously, identifying what is important, ignoring what is not, and facilitating their arousal when needed.

While we close our eyes and turn our sight inward, our senses of hearing and smell appear to remain somewhat intact while we sleep. From an evolutionary perspective, retaining the ability to smell smoke or to hear approaching animals, footsteps, or cries for help would be essential for survival. I never cease to be amazed by the fact that when I set my alarm to wake up early, I inevitably open my eyes a few minutes before it rings. While I sleep away the night, some thread of consciousness that knows how much I hate rude awakenings keeps track of time, remembers when I have to get up, and awakens me at just the right moment.

It appears there are many gradations in the continuum between sleeping and waking realities. As we slip between the two, we cannot help but trail residues from one to the other, for each bears a touch of the other. Our concerns by day often take the stage in our dreams, just as the feelings that occupy us at night sometimes stay with us long after we open our eyes. There are even times when "a dream haunts us and compels our attention during the day," noted nineteenth-century psychologist William James, "figuring in our consciousness as a sort of subuniverse alongside of the waking world."

Unseen Collaborators

Several years ago, I went to visit someone who lived a few hours away from my home. The drive involved taking a narrow dirt road that wound down the side of a steep canyon and back up the other side. I had been that way before and seen the rusted-out and picked-over carcasses of cars that had gone over the edge and tumbled down into the canyon. The night before, I dreamed that I was driving that road, rounding a blind corner, when a car suddenly appeared from the opposite direction. I turned to avoid it, lost control of my car, and went over the side of the canyon.

The nightmare worried me the next morning, mostly because I rarely dream of something I am planning to do the next day. I considered taking a longer, circuitous way to avoid the canyon, but I love that gorge and wanted to see the river that runs through it, so I left early instead. By the time I started down into the canyon, I had forgotten about the dream. I was singing along to my favorite CD with my windows open when a bee darted into my car. Believing I was allergic to bees at the time, I whipped my head around to watch where it went and did not see the car coming toward me until it was upon me. I braked, as did the other driver, swerved, and… we skated right by each other, spitting gravel all the while. Later, when I stopped at the river to catch my breath, I remembered my dream.

What interests me about this experience is that it displays a conversation that occurred between conscious and unconscious—waking and dreaming—parts of me. My daytime nervousness about the drive probably sparked my fearsome dream, which in turn prompted me to leave early and drive more slowly. Since things turned out well, I like to think the dialogue saved me, but it may just have reminded me of what I already knew but was tempted to ignore.

If we dream repeatedly of banging on a locked door, we are more apt to stop struggling against something that will not budge, or turn around and try another approach, in the days to come without ever realizing the connection between our dreaming and waking lives. More often than not, there is an emotion—in my case, fear of an accident—that connects those parallel worlds, running like a wormhole between them. There may even be an image that both tells the story and evokes the emotions in one fell swoop, one that functions as the crux of the dream, the hub of its dizzying wheel, the still point of its devastating insight.

This invisible, surreptitious communication between waking and sleeping worlds probably occurs more than we realize. As John Steinbeck once noted, "It is a common experience that a problem difficult at night is resolved in the morning after the committee of sleep has worked on it."[9] When friends advise us to sleep on an important decision, they imply that we do our best when we allow both our sleeping and waking minds to weigh in on a given situation. Creative people often come to rely upon the intelligence of this unconscious processing. Scottish novelist Robert Louis Stevenson described "unseen collaborators" within him "who do one-half my work while I am fast asleep, and in all human likelihood, do the rest for me as well, when I am wide awake and fondly suppose I do it myself."

Stevenson's words were remarkably prescient. In recent decades, cognitive psychologists have discovered that most mental processing occurs unconsciously both by day and by night. While we focus on what is in front of us at the moment, our unconscious minds work automatically to collect and process huge amounts of information that are too hidden, too abundant, or too complex for us to notice at the time. This nonconscious mind, as cognitive psychologists call it, scans continuously for meaningful patterns in everything around us.[10] It enables us to hear someone say our names across a crowded room or recall a movie title we have forgotten hours later. When we rely on a hunch to make a decision, we are placing our trust in this offline processing.

While the nonconscious mind works day and night, sleep may take us closer to that subterranean sea of information, that subuniverse, as James calls it, which lies alongside our waking world. The more we learn about the interpenetration of waking and sleeping states, the more it seems that we are continually sliding along a continuum between the two and are never fully established in one or the other. Like the yin-yang symbol, each contains a bit of the other as we cycle through stages of more or less alertness throughout our twenty-four-hour day.

Psychologist and dream researcher Rosalind Cartwright speaks of the twenty-four-hour mind to emphasize that our brains never shut down.[11] They just shift gears. Henry Ward Beecher put it more poetically in the nineteenth century: "We sleep, but the loom of life never stops, and the pattern which was weaving when the sun went down is weaving when it comes up in the morning."

10

THE INVISIBLE LABORS OF SLEEP: MEMORY AND INVENTION

My seven-year-old stepdaughter, Lauren, stood in her Batwoman pajamas next to her bed waiting for me. It was bedtime, and the room was dark except for the tiny glowing stars we had glued to the ceiling. I pulled back the covers, and Lauren started to crawl into her night nest of pillows, stuffed animals, hair ribbons, and glitter that surrounded her in sleep, night after night, arranged and rearranged by her somnolent stirrings. Then, as if struck by a sudden insight, Lauren spun around and cried: "Why do we have to go to sleep?"

That question has circled and hounded the field of sleep science like buzzards over roadkill for many years. However, the question strikes me as an odd one. Do we ask ourselves: why watch sunsets or scratch mosquito bites? Is not the answer obvious? Because we want to and cannot keep ourselves from doing it. Every living creature partakes in the activity of sleep in one form or another. The fact that the question continues to be asked reflects our collective disregard for the time we spend asleep, what psychologist Rubin R. Naiman has termed our wake-centric cultural bias. After all, do we ever ask why we have to wake up?[1]

Sleep researchers now state with confidence that sleep is not just a simple pleasure or guilty indulgence; it is necessary for our cognitive, physical, and emotional well-being. In fact, they are filling the airwaves with justifications for something that is clearly in need of defending, something that appears to be headed toward extinction as we speak. The first benefit that was proven beyond a doubt was that sleep improves memory and cognitive performance—a perfect first line of defense in a world that values productivity over almost everything else.

Memory and Learning

In the 1990s, neuroscientist Matthew Walker and his associates began monitoring the firing of neurons in the memory centers of the brains of four pink-eared, black-and-white laboratory rats.[2] A computer translated their neuronal firings into sharp, staccato crackling sounds while the rats learned a circular maze to get chocolate-flavored sprinkles. Every time a rat ran the maze, the crackles sounded in a distinct, identifiable sequence.

Then, one day, when one of the rats had eaten enough sprinkles and fallen fast asleep, Walker made a remarkable discovery. The sequence of crackles the rat produced when learning the maze repeated—in the same order, only twenty times faster—during brief bursts of electrical activity called ripples, which overlay the huge, slow waves of deep sleep. It appeared that this rat was replaying his memory of the maze in compressed time, as if practicing this newly learned skill in fast-forward, and the correlation was so exact, Walker and his associates were able to tell what part of the maze was being reviewed. It was the first clear neurological evidence that mammals revisit important daytime learning during SW sleep.

Walker's rats were also better at running their mazes after they slept. In fact, the amount of their improvement was proportional to the length of time spent reactivating the maze memory in SW sleep. People are no different than rodents on this score. We too improve our abilities to perform tasks and remember significant events and facts after an interval of sleep, which has prompted researchers to recommend that students take naps while studying. In turn, sleep deprivation impairs learning and memory, reducing our capacities to form new connections between brain cells.

Years ago, a piano teacher suggested I take time off my daily practice periodically because, as she said, "for some reason, people play better after they've slept a night or two." Her observation was shared by the Roman orator Quintilian many centuries before, who noted that: "[It] is a curious fact, of which the reason is not obvious, that the interval of a single night will greatly increase the strength of the memory." Now my piano teacher's casual observation is backed by scientific research. Studies reveal that learning improves over the course of several nights without any practice.[3] In fact, sleep provides the equivalent of twice as much practice. We are smarter when we wake up than when we went to bed.

Most researchers agree that short-term memory is anchored and translated into long-term memory when we sleep. The process, called memory consolidation, appears to involve two simultaneous procedures: weakening rarely used neural connections and strengthening the patterns of newly formed memories by replaying them. Neuroscientist Mayank Mehta likened it to erasing the chalkboard so new messages do not overlap and get confused with old ones.[4] Giulio Tononi and his colleague Chiara Cirelli at the University of Wisconsin–Madison propose that the large, slow waves that dominate SW sleep wash the board clean by reducing the number of active connections, while the brief bursts of faster activity, called ripples, inscribe new learning.[5] They work together to enable new memories to stand out clearly. It seems that we forget in order to remember, and we do this best when we are deeply asleep, all is quiet, our breathing is slow, and the slate is clean.

Memory in REM Sleep

REM sleep performs another, equally important job in handling memory, according to a theory proposed by two prominent research psychiatrists, Robert Stickgold and Matthew Walker.[6] While SW sleep preserves individual memories with relative accuracy, REM sleep assimilates these memories into what is already known. This requires several steps: extracting the gist of what was learned, connecting it to related memories, and filing it away in existing networks of knowledge, or schemas, for further use. The process has been likened to that of a change sorter separating coins into different slots for storage. Memories are distilled into familiar topics—like French grammar or the way a family pet behaves—bundled into readable chunks, and filed away for further use. In the process, we begin to infer the big picture from disparate pieces of information.

How our minds and brains decide what is worth remembering, what to call it, and where to put it is not clear, but many think emotions play an important role.[7] Some experiences are seared into our memory while others fade away, and the difference between the two appears to lie with the level of emotional significance. Events that threaten our survival, like the death of a loved one, a major rejection, or a natural disaster, are highlighted by the presence of adrenaline, and they stick with us, even if we wish they did not. Ecstatic experiences, be it the birth of a baby or a religious conversion, also marked by intense emotion, find room in our memory banks as well. But the cars you see on your way to work do not—unless one of them runs into you. The heightened emotional and physiological arousal of REM sleep appears to tag the salient memories, making them easier to retrieve later, while ignoring the rest.

Recent memories are also replayed in REM sleep, as they are in SW sleep. However, they are repeated in a fractured, jumbled arrangement. "When we're awake," explains psychologist and dream researcher Rosalind Cartwright, "we're used to thinking in a logical, linear way, one thing leading to the next in a straightforward line. But dreams are constructed more like Scotch plaids, with recent memory placed on top of earlier memories, all linked by feeling, not logic."[8] Like collage artists, our brains work quickly and intuitively in REM sleep, without the constraints of reason or the corrections of exact recall to connect, overlay, and blend recent memories with past ones, including those gathered by our nonconscious minds while we were busy elsewhere. The *Aranyaka Upanishad* offers a beautiful description: "When one goes to sleep, he takes along the material of this all-containing world, himself tears it apart, himself builds it up, and dreams by his own brightness."

Researchers call these intuitive leaps free association—the same term Freud used for the technique he developed to access the internal logic of dreams—and they typically follow along the lines of emotional resemblance, knitting similar memories together. Artemidorus, a second century Mid-Eastern dream interpreter, called this associational style the "juxtaposition of similarities."[9] Some of our dreams may actually display the complex webs of emotionally toned similarities we have woven over the course of a lifetime.

Psychiatrist Robert Stickgold conducted an interesting study that demonstrated this intuitive, associational style of memory integration.[10] It involved showing participants a list of medical terms and later asking them if the word hospital was on the list. (It wasn't.) Those who had REM sleep before answering were much more likely to (wrongly) answer yes than those who did not. Researchers surmised that when the medical terms were filed into existing memory banks during REM sleep, they were inadvertently associated with the word *hospital*, perhaps because we are likely to hear those words in a hospital, and hospital visits tend to be emotional, for better or worse. This study also hints at some of the distortions that can occur when memories are assimilated. Like immigrants in a new country, recent memories drop accents and smooth over distinctions in order to fit in to the existing order—our storehouse of past experience. It may also explain, in part, why witnesses to the same event may remember it differently.

The process of making and integrating memories enables us to extract lessons from the past to prepare for future challenges. These lessons are more than mere records of experience. When connected with existing networks of knowledge, they become the very beliefs that define who we are and who we are going to be. Every time an association is made, something is learned, memory is altered, knowledge is refined, and pre-existing beliefs are usually, though not always, confirmed. It is the essence of brain plasticity and, apparently, one of the jobs REM sleep performs. The more we learn by day, the longer we spend in REM sleep that night.

As the night progresses through successive cycles of SW and REM sleep, new learning is repeated and assimilated into ever-widening nets of increasingly remote and original associations. Dreams become longer, more complicated, and farther reaching. They play out what could have happened but did not, pose alternative scenarios to make right what went wrong, and bring more information to bear on the places we get stuck. In the morning, we are left with memories that are a little less accurate but more meaningful, accessible, and useful.

Creative Solutions

We also emerge from sleep with improved capacities for creative problem solving. As researchers Matthew Walker and Jeffrey Ellenbogen explained, "You go to bed with pieces of the memory puzzle, and awaken with the jigsaw completed."[11] Louis Agassiz, the nineteenth-century biologist, did just that.[12] He was struggling to visualize the shape and features of an ancient fish from a single, partial fossil, and he dreamed that he saw the fish before him two nights in a row, but he could not remember the images well enough in the morning to sketch them out. On the third night, he put a paper and pencil under his pillow and waited for the dream to return. When it did, he drew his vision in the dark, half asleep. The next morning he realized that his dream drawing satisfied the requirements of the fossil in a way he could not imagine awake.

There are times like this when sleep literally offers the solution we have been seeking; but, more often than not, it simply primes our minds to be able to arrive at the answer ourselves. The nineteenth-century French professor Hervey de Saint-Denys, who recorded, illustrated, and interpreted thousands of his own dreams, noticed that the dreaming mind often considers a problem by means of an internal debate, or dialogue, with itself, assuming varied stances to develop a wider perspective.[13] At other times, he added, the dreaming mind superimposes images to dissolve apparent dichotomies and contradictions. It is like working a jigsaw puzzle, turning the pieces around, trying to fit them into empty spaces, laying them on top of others.

The ancient Greeks had a metaphoric way of describing the unconscious processes of memory formation, one that not only honored what was forgotten but also recognized its relationship to creative inspiration.[14] They explained that everyone who falls asleep—or dies—must surrender his or her memories to the running waters of Lethe ("forgetting" or "oblivion") in the Underworld. But those recollections did not disappear; instead, they soaked into the earth, where they were sifted and sorted. In time, they re-emerged in the rippling waters of Mnemosyne ("memory"), where the residues of lived-out lives floated like flecks of fine sand at the bottom of her bubbling spring. That is where the Muses of artistic and scientific invention could be found. In the paradoxical elegance of ancient Greek thought, the past experiences of all people fueled future inspiration once digested by the earth, our dreaming bodies.

The process of sifting, sorting, and digesting memories often requires that the emotional charge attached to them—the sticky, muddling sorrows, angers, and regrets—be stripped away to reveal the clear outlines of truth. Then, and only then, can our future selves make use of them. In this way, sleep works to restore emotional equilibrium and foster understanding. "There, that is our secret: go to sleep!" wrote Robert Browning, "You will wake, and remember, and understand."

11

KNITTING UP THE "RAVELED SLEAVE OF CARE": EMOTIONAL RESTORATION

I was running as fast as I could down the mountainside, but the Wicked Witch of the West from *The Wizard of Oz* was right behind me, her black cape and hair flying behind her in the wind, driving a bright red convertible, top down. It was inevitable: the witch would catch me, and I would be done for. This is the earliest dream I remember, and it prompted the only time that I remember charging into my parents' bedroom screaming and waking them to comfort me. More than two thousand years ago, the Greek philosopher Aristotle described dreams as "echoes of emotionally charged sense-perceptions from daily life."[1] While I do not recall what happened the day before my nightmare, I do remember the thrill and terror I felt every year I watched the famous movie on television with my siblings, each of us frozen in our spots on the carpet in front of the big black box.

Sleep researchers have begun to confirm Aristotle's notion that we carry the emotional concerns of our days into our nights. As Shakespeare noted, sleep "knits up the raveled sleave of care."

That may seem obvious to many, but the emerging consensus has evoked a renaissance in scientific thinking about the role that sleep and dreams play in managing the emotions that get the better of us by day. Not long ago, many scientists believed that dreams were nonsense, vestigial "by-products" of sleep, "random firings" of a nervous system in sleep mode, something like the screen savers on our computers, or the feeble attempts of our forebrains to make sense out of those firings.[2]

People who monitor their dreams often note that they have a way of picking up on passing anxieties from the previous day and enlarging them, as if placing them under a microscope.[3] Veiled criticisms, near disasters, and offhand comments we may have overlooked at the time are evoked through emotion-laden images and matched with older memories, at times revealing unseen patterns. Occasionally, we wake understanding something that eluded us the night before—that someone has been lying to us, for instance, or it's time to get our blood sugar levels checked. As the Bulgarian author Elias Canetti allegedly once noted: "All the things one has forgotten scream for help in dreams."

Furthermore, sleep selectively recalls the emotionally arousing incidents of our days over the neutral, matter-of-fact ones.[4] The arousal of our fight-or-flight sympathetic nervous systems apparently marks these experiences for review. From this fact alone, it would seem that our dreaming brains just make things worse by focusing on the negative. However, subsequent rounds of REM sleep over the course of one or several nights usually function to reduce the visceral autonomic charge that accompanies these frightening or enraging experiences, helping us to put them to rest.

Rosalind Cartwright followed the dreams of twenty recently divorced men and women, half of whom met the criteria for depression, over five months. She discovered that those who recovered best remembered more dreams, and their dreams were longer and more complex, often integrating fragments of recent emotional experiences with older ones. They also made a gradual shift over time from playing more passive roles in their dreams to more active ones. Their dreams, noted Cartwright, were "like a rehearsal for recovery." Those who did not improve had shorter, more static dreams or no recall at all. While it may seem obvious to people who make a habit of attending to their dreams, Cartwright's study was the first scientific investigation to demonstrate that the content of our dreams, not just their occurrence, plays an important role in our recovery from emotional trauma.[5]

In light of Cartwright's research and neurological studies, psychiatrist Mathew Walker proposed in 2009 that REM sleep functions like "overnight therapy" to strip the charge from salient memories through repeated reiterations while retaining the essential learning.[6] He called it the "sleep to forget [the emotion] and sleep to remember [the lesson]" model of cognitive and emotional processing, adding that sleep is uniquely qualified to accomplish the task. REM sleep, in particular, is the only time during our days and nights when our levels of norepinephrine, a kind of adrenaline, plummet, reducing arousal. In this way, the charged schemas, or beliefs, by which we stake our lives, and of which we may not be consciously aware, are routinely worked and reworked, unraveled and rewoven whenever current events activate them. Our sense of self in the world is continually updated, for better or for worse. It may take one night, several nights, or even years of shuttling back and forth between REM and SW sleep to take the sting out of the most disturbing experiences, but we usually come to greater understanding and detachment.

Double Consciousness

How REM sleep strips the emotional charge from our memories remains a mystery. The repetitions and revisions themselves may do the trick. After all, the more often we tell a story from our lives, the more detached we (usually) feel from it, and the more capable we are of understanding what happened in a larger context. The frequent changes and multiple perspectives of our dreams may also play a role. As our emotions twist and turn with every switch of scene and characters, we come to experience many, if not all, sides of an issue. For example, in a dream about a lost child, there may be the eagerly exploring youngster who becomes a frightened little boy and the frantic, searching mother peering down streets, a growling dog, the ornate ironwork of the park bench under which the child hides from the dog, and the teeth that melt into a silver coin. Far away and close up, the lost and the looking, the straight and the curving, the conceivable and the inconceivable, all offer different perspectives, new orientations, that inch us closer to emotional resolution.

When I started this book, I promised myself that I would not recount many personal dreams, even though they comprise the most memorable part of sleep, because dreams feel like they wither and dry up when torn from their roots in the life of an individual, a culture, and a time. However, the following dream illustrates how sleep can change our feelings and thoughts so well, I couldn't resist. The dream came to me years ago, when I was co-chair of a neighborhood organization that had become embroiled in a contentious public battle over a proposed development. As one who prefers to avoid conflict, I found my role of fighting for one side against the other painfully uncomfortable, so much so that I felt sick to my stomach most of the time. Then I had this dream: I was floating out in space, looking down at the Earth with a detached curiosity, when I zoomed in on a particular place where a spectacular Shakespearean drama was occurring. Suddenly, I was sucked down onto the stage and into the body of one of the actors, knowing that my job was to play this role to the best of my ability so that the others could play theirs and the drama could proceed to its conclusion.

I woke up feeling that it was okay, even appropriate, to take a side in the fight, realizing that all of us, even those watching from afar, would learn from the experience. I also understood that my opponents were just like me, neither good nor bad, simply actors doing their jobs. My dream offered what Ralph Waldo Emerson termed the "double consciousness" of sleep, one that is both subjective and objective. As a result, my sense of self became more fluid, adaptable, and inclusive. In her study of dream interpretation in late antiquity, Patricia Cox Miller likened the effect of dreaming to the "twist of a kaleidoscope; the pieces of a life's experience throw themselves together in a new pattern, a new way of picturing, or visualizing, one's self."[7] When dreams offer up these multiple perspectives, sleep has the potential to massage our hearts and minds, helping us to change in ways that seemed impossible the night before.

When people do not get enough sleep, this process of emotional recalibration gets interrupted, especially because most of our REM sleep occurs later in the night, during the hours that tend to get cut short. Studies demonstrate that sleep-deprived people are more likely to respond to negative cues, ignore positive ones, and react impulsively and aggressively.[8] They become more rigid mentally and emotionally, displaying knee-jerk reactions rather than thoughtful responses.[9] As a friend of mine says, "Without enough sleep, we turn into two-year-olds."

There is growing evidence that insomnia can create and/or exasperate existing emotional problems and that emotional difficulties can interfere with sleep, fueling a vicious cycle of negative effects with potentially disastrous results.[10] Those who commit suicide often have a history of insomnia.[11] Even good sleepers experience more anxiety after a night of no sleep; those predisposed to worry can develop full-blown anxiety disorders from poor sleep.[12] If the "best bridge between despair and hope is a good night's sleep," as American entrepreneur and marketing guru E. Joseph Cossman allegedly said, then we are in trouble without it. We need our dreaming time, day and night, to soothe our ruffled feathers and restore emotional equilibrium. Life has a way of pushing our buttons; sleep may serve, in part, to reset them. Parents know this. When their children are tired and upset, they tuck them into bed and say, "Let's talk about it in the morning." Perhaps this is what the Dalai Lama meant when he called sleep "the best meditation."[13]

"A Dream, a Nightmare, a Madness"

However, there are times, especially after life-threatening trauma, when we wake from sleep worse off than when we went to bed, having endured horrific nightmares, night terrors, dangerous bouts of sleepwalking, or an inability to sleep for fear of these experiences. The hypervigilance that often follows trauma fragments and disrupts sleep, undermining its restorative effect. The process of emotional recalibration seems to falter, and each subsequent stage of REM dreaming can reignite and perpetuate the fear and helplessness, often leading to chronic insomnia.[14]

Sleeplessness may be the body's first line of defense against trauma, as extended wakefulness improves the functioning of the neurotransmitter serotonin and dampens the cortisol-driven stress response, both of which are implicated in post-traumatic stress, while higher levels of ATP boost mood.[15] Maintaining wakefulness for the first several hours after a traumatic event may even reduce the risk of developing long-term post-traumatic stress.[16] Many people have accidently discovered, and research has demonstrated, that staying up all night can relieve depression, but only until the next sleep.[17] Delaying sleep after a trauma is probably a good instinct in the short run, but it does not help in the long run because it deprives us of the sleep we need to integrate experience and function well.

Nightmares at such times are more like flashbacks, in that they literally replay pieces of the traumatic event with little change over time, like the repetitive play that many traumatized children perform. REM sleep comes sooner and stays longer, while recuperative SW sleep shortens, disrupting the delicate homeostatic cycles of sleep.[18] Benzodiazepines, commonly prescribed for intractable insomnia, perpetuate the trend by further reducing restorative SW sleep.[19] The newer nonbenzodiazepines, such as Ambien, Lunesta, and Sonata, do not restrict SW sleep but may pose other problems. Preliminary research conducted by psychologist Sara C. Mednick at the University of California, Riverside, revealed that Ambien heightens the recollection of, and reaction to, negative memories, but not positive ones.[20] When sleep is broken by nightmares, people wake feeling exhausted, as if they have been fighting a war all night, which they have, in a sense. They get touchier and more reactive by day, focusing on negative cues and ignoring positive ones, thereby ensuring that the war will continue the next night.

Repetitive, unchanging nightmares reflect and perpetuate a train of negative consequences. This vicious cycle of defensive hypervigilance can lead to serious depression and despair without intervention. Dostoevsky knew it well when he wrote: "A dream, a nightmare, a madness." The link between insomnia, nightmares, and mood disorders has become so strong since the turn of the twenty-first century; some observers have suggested that sleep deprivation may play a key role in the initiation and perpetuation of the major mood disorders.[21] Studies also reveal that insomnia usually precedes episodes of depression by about five weeks. Moreover, the reduction in SW sleep and the increase in REM intensity and duration are closely correlated with the severity of depression. The effects of sleep disruption on mood, perception, and behavior are so strong that patients are sometimes misdiagnosed with psychiatric disorders when they simply need better sleep.[22]

Many antidepressants reduce REM sleep duration and intensity, and some observers suggest that this restoration of more balanced sleep may be the primary means by which they work, when they do. Even if a causal link does not exist, our mental health and mood stability require that the cruel cycle of inadequate sleep, distorted thought, and emotional volatility be broken so that sleep can do its job of restoration.

Sleepwalking

People who get little SW sleep are more prone to sleepwalking, especially if it runs in the family, if they are young, or if they are under stress or the influence of alcohol or certain drugs. Many of these factors converge to arouse someone from deep SW sleep; once they are up, they are awake enough to move about, but not awake enough to be aware of, or responsible for, what they are doing. Observers often note that they seem to look right through them, move like zombies, and do not respond to intervention.

Usually, they do ordinary things, like go to the bathroom or get a snack, but they can also do dangerous things, like cook or drive. Since the prefrontal cortex, which monitors and controls our impulses, is disengaged in SW sleep, instinctual drives for food, sex, escape, or self-defense take over, prompting sleepwalkers to eat everything in the fridge, engage in inappropriate sex, fight off hallucinated attackers, even jump out of windows.

On rare occasions, sleepwalkers have committed murder and suicide. Neuroscientists testifying in their defense in court have explained that we are not conscious and capable of considered action when we are sleepwalking.[23] These and other cases of neurological impairment raise serious moral and legal questions, undermining western assumptions of free will and responsibility. Are we really capable of making sound decisions at all times? Neuroscientist David Eagleman has proposed a radical change in jurisprudence, from a focus on the defendant's culpability (did he do it?) to his capacity (will he do it again?).[24] Cases of sleepwalking, along with brain injuries and tumors, may begin to set precedents for a sea change in Western attitudes and law.

There was a time in my life when I had nightmares every night for a month. It started after someone I admired and trusted accused me of lying. I was upset at first, but not devastated, until the nightmares started. Versions of the same scenario—someone trying to kill me because I told an unforgivable truth—played out every night, inevitably thrusting me out of sleep in a sweat, shot through with adrenaline, after which I usually spent the rest of the night awake, fuming over the incident. I rarely got a full night's sleep, and by the end of the month, this relatively minor incident had come to assume mammoth proportions in my life. I trembled with rage by day, wanted everyone around me to take my side, and felt their unwillingness to get involved to be a denial of my very existence. My nightmares became self-fulfilling prophecies.

Clearly, the incident triggered something bigger in me, probably an underlying schema that subtly—or not so subtly—colored my perceptions. But the nightmares were not helping. They were making things worse by exaggerating my faulty thinking and emotional reactivity to the point of derangement.

I wish someone had been able to explain to me the importance of getting good sleep, especially when we are triggered, and how the lack of it can distort thought and inflate negative emotions. When nightmares repeat the same thing over and over rather than change with time, something needs to be done to reclaim the restorative balance between REM and SW sleep. It cannot be a coincidence that nightmares wake us up while other dreams drift downstream in the waters of forgetting while we sleep. They call for our attention, as if waving a red flag or ringing an alarm, and require a waking response. Almost every culture provides ways to address the disturbance that nightmares reflect and inflame, be it changing sleep arrangements, performing ceremony to release negative energies, receiving acupuncture to balance pulses, seeking guidance from dream interpreters, or taking antidepressants to reduce REM sleep and increase SW sleep.

The famed Belgian comic book artist known as Hergé, who wrote the popular *Tintin* series between 1958 until his death in 1983, was plagued by nightmares of whiteness during an intensely troubling crisis in his life.[25] When he consulted a Swiss psychoanalyst who encouraged him to stop working, Hergé responded by immersing himself in creating what many consider to be his best book: *Tintin in Tibet*, which takes place in the all-white snow-covered Himalayas. By the time he finished the book, the nightmares had vanished. The eighteenth-century Scottish philosopher Thomas Reid stopped years of nightmares by repeatedly telling himself that the dreams were not real and could not hurt him.[26] In ancient Greece, dreamers told bad dreams to the sun in the understanding that sunlight breaks spells and disperses the demons of darkness.[27] Ancient Mesopotamians told their nightmares to lumps of clay and then threw them into the river, reciting: "As I throw you into the water, you will crumble and disintegrate, and may the evil consequences of all the dreams soon be gone, melted away, and be many miles removed from my body."[28] Each approach, in its own way, tries to get the train back on its track, the soul back on its path, and sleep back into its own rhythm.

In therapeutic circles, some counselors have begun to teach people to change their nightmares in their imaginations by imagining new endings until the nightmares resolve. This practice, called image rehearsal therapy, rests on the discovery that imagined experience is real experience to the brain.[29] This technique reminds me of times when, as a child forensic interviewer, I have heard children report horrific abuse with convincing detail and emotion only to tack on a fantastic, implausible ending to recover from the telling. One eleven-year-old boy told me he took a sword out of his pajamas and cut off his uncle's head. Sometimes the imagined response is believable but untrue. A seven-year-old girl confided that she told the policeman next door what happened and he promised to stop it. Investigators rushed to find the officer who could possibly serve as a witness for the prosecution only to discover there was no policeman next door and never had been. There seems to be an innate human need to revise negative experiences to restore a sense of self as strong and capable.

That need is usually evident in the course that most repetitive nightmares take over time of their own accord. Psychiatrist Ernest Hartmann has observed a typical progression in recurring nightmares.[30] At first, the content changes somewhat, but the feeling remains. One night it is your house on fire; the next night, it is a tidal wave about to engulf you. Either way, there is the sense of imminent destruction. Or you've forgotten your children on the train one night, and you cannot reach a drowning man the next, feeling guilty both times. Gradually, when sleep is able to do its job, the dreams begin to incorporate more of our life experiences, the images become less literal and more symbolic, and the emotions get smaller and more tolerable. There is a shift from helplessness to active participation. Eventually, other dreams arise, often including pieces of the nightmares, but in a context that defuses them. The nightmares fade away, losing their charge and frequency unless triggered by another trauma.

Ally, Adversary, or Both?

There are some nightmares that accompany us through life, as if prodding us to do what we must. Former US President Lyndon Johnson reported to his biographer, Doris Kearns Goodwin, that he had recurring nightmares of paralysis at critical points in his life.[31] When Johnson was five years old, he dreamed repeatedly of sitting in a chair in the middle of an open field, unable to move, with a herd of cattle stampeding toward him. The dreams came back after his heart attack when he was forty-six, only that time he was chained to the chair in his office, unable to leave work. When he was serving as vice president, he dreamed repeatedly that he was lying paralyzed in the Red Room of the White House. Johnson told Goodwin that whenever he had the dream, he would get up, walk through the White House until he found the portrait of Woodrow Wilson, whose stroke effectively ended his presidency, and touch it. The last set of nightmares occurred in 1968, when Johnson was president and the Vietnam War had come to a standstill. In these dreams, he was swimming in a river, unable to reach the shore because he was going in circles and getting nowhere. Johnson told Goodwin that the dream helped him to make the decision to forgo running for re-election and to focus, instead, on ending the war. There were no more nightmares after that.

It seems a contradiction that such a powerful man would be haunted by nightmares of being paralyzed and not getting anywhere; yet dreams have a way of encompassing oppositions. Perhaps they spurred him on, motivating him to assume power and make difficult decisions. Maybe they reminded him of his mortality, pushing him to step down when the time called for it. Regardless, it appears that this string of nightmares was an invisible player in the course of Johnson's life, reflecting his predicaments and steering his decisions, extracting moments of wisdom from years of suffering.

It's an age-old process, one that Aeschylus, the Greek playwright who wrote around the time the *Upanishads* were being completed, described well when he wrote: "He who learns must suffer. And even in our sleep pain that cannot forget falls drop by drop upon the heart, and in our own despair, against our will, comes wisdom to us by the awful grace of God." Sleep can be subversive in this way. It owes no allegiance to our waking selves nor to the larger societal powers that be.

12

SLEEP HAS NO MASTER: SUBVERSIVE DREAMING

When I was in my thirties, trying to catch up on sleep after a demanding semester of graduate school, a strange thing happened. In the still, gray hours before dawn, when it feels as if the earth itself has drawn in a long, slow breath and paused, I heard someone call my name. I opened my eyes. An ashen gray sky cast a dim, diffused light across the far side of the room, and it took me a few moments to realize that no one was there. Even so, I knew who had called for me: my uncle Abe.

Uncle Abe was in a coma at the time, having suffered a heart attack the night he entered a rehabilitation unit in the local hospital a few months before. I didn't actually see him; I just felt his presence, as if he were in the room with me. The enormous weight I had always felt around him, as a large man of great accomplishments and devastating flaws, was miraculously lifted. In an instant of recognition, he let me know that he was free and I was not to blame.

I believe I was awake at the time, but I am not certain. What I can say with confidence is that the experience rose out of my sleep, and I suspect it could not have come at any other time because the outside world is so captivating when I am up and about. Sleep removes us from the continuous barrage of sensory input that commands our attention by day and cocoons us in a world of subtle, inwardly felt impressions. In Taoist terms, our attention shifts from the dense physical body to the subtle energy body.[1] The New Guinea Asabano, like many indigenous people, say that the bonds between our bodies and our souls are unbuttoned in sleep, allowing us to penetrate the thin curtain that ordinarily keeps us apart from the spiritual world.[2] The fourteenth-century Muslim scholar Ibn Kaldun went so far as to claim that God gave sleep to humans so that we could glimpse the truth behind the veil created by our external senses.[3] In the cautious parlance of contemporary science, sleep enables specialized cognitive processes.

I have no way of knowing for sure whether my uncle actually came to my bedside in some form or if I imagined him there out of some unknown need of my own. This uncertainty about the nature and origin of sleep experiences has dogged humanity for millennia, invoking a slew of existential questions: Do we separate from our slumbering bodies to roam the world at night? Or do we imagine and emit these world-embedded stories we call dreams like sparks from a fire for reasons we don't understand—or for no reason at all? Do we have one self or many selves? Do we inhabit one world or many worlds? Are dreams true or false, neither or both? As anthropologist Waud H. Kracke observed: "Dreams are the most obstinate stumbling block to our secure knowledge that we 'know' the world around us."[4]

Our Common Heritage as Dreamers

The first time a friend told me he did not dream, I was stupefied, as if he had confessed he had never ridden a bike, chewed gum, or partaken in some other everyday activity. With time, I came to feel a mixture of envy and sorrow for people who do not have dreams. On the one hand, life would be simpler, more coherent and reliable, if we were not subject to the nightly scramblings and intrusions of other realities. On the other hand, it would seem so small and flat without them. Some of the most stunning experiences of my life have occurred under the cover of sleep.

When scientists began investigating sleep seriously in the second half of the twentieth century by monitoring college students sleeping overnight in their labs, they discovered something interesting.[5] Students who insisted they did not dream usually reported dreamlike sequences when they were woken during REM sleep; they just did not remember them come morning. It happened so consistently, researchers concluded that everybody dreams four to six times a night. Since then, researchers have identified a few conditions that may prevent dreaming; however, the basic claim remains true. Human beings are innately dreaming creatures.

We are not the only animals who dream, of course. When our cats paw at the air while napping and our dogs whimper and wiggle their legs in their sleep, we know intuitively that they are dreaming, perhaps of catching birds or chasing rabbits. Now, with the technological ability to record neuronal firing patterns in small clusters of brain cells, scientists have shown that we are not projecting our experiences onto our pets. They have demonstrated that zebra finches dream of singing, and lab mice dream of repeating the mazes they run by day to get tasty treats.[6] Gorillas who have learned sign language have even described dream experiences to their human friends.[7] Our penchant for dreaming has been retained throughout our evolution as human beings. We stood up, lost body hair, and changed skin color, but we kept—and perhaps enhanced—our capacity to slip in and out of dreaming states on a regular basis.

Our brains are wondrously adept at moving between states of waking, sleeping, and dreaming repeatedly during the course of our days and nights, relying upon complex, carefully orchestrated sequences of electrochemical signals to activate and deactivate parts of our neural circuitry. Consciousness comes and goes in the process, and it cannot always keep the thread of what was just happening when shifting states. Some people are better at holding on to the baffling flux of feeling and imagery we call dreams upon waking. The talent—or liability, depending upon your perspective—to remember one's dreams has been variously attributed to personality style, length of sleep, manner of awakening, attitude toward dreams, and intensity of the dreams themselves.

However, even those without the natural aptitude can cultivate it, in much the same way we learn any skill: preparation and practice. Throughout history, people in a wide variety of cultures have developed ways to induce, or incubate, dreams using prayer, ceremony, and purifying rituals.[8] In the ancient Mediterranean, seekers bathed in natural springs, fasted, made offerings to the gods, and slept in holy temples to invite healing dreams. Dream incubation, as it was called, continued well into the Christian era when people slept in churches on the tombs of the saints. On the North American continent, native peoples from many of the Plains tribes conducted vision quests involving fasting, praying, and sleeping in sacred places to obtain assistance from their dreams, just as their ancestors had done for centuries. Central American Mayans slept in dream houses where they could make contact with Nahuales, ancestral spirit guides.[9]

Research indicates that, on average, we forget 50 percent of what we dream within the first five minutes after waking and 90 percent after ten minutes.[10] If we use an alarm to wake up, get out of bed immediately, or do not get enough sleep, more is lost. Sleep debt—the accumulation of sleep lost over the course of days or weeks—is the most common and effective dream thief because it steals the later hours of sleep when most of our dreams occur. To improve recall, experts recommend that we go to bed in time to get enough sleep and then remind ourselves as we fall asleep to remember our dreams in the morning. Upon waking, it is best to lie still, notice any feelings, images, or sensations (no matter how small or insignificant), write them down immediately, and reflect upon them later. The key is to pay attention to the dim traces of our nightly adventures still with us the moment we open our eyes. The more interest we take in our dreams, the more we remember.

The Inalienable Right to Dream

Dreams are free and equally available to the rich and poor, young and old, addled and adept, free and incarcerated. Like weeds that poke through cement, they will sprout in any soil, against any resistance. There is no malicious government or tyrant that can outlaw dreams or take them away from us, as Synesius of Cyrene observed in the fifth century AD. Even though they have been maligned as the work of the devil in some eras and dismissed as nonsense in others, people around the world have continued to cherish dreaming, perhaps because it is the only place we are truly free. As the popular Jamaican slave proverb notes: "Sleep hab no massa" (Sleep has no master). In that innermost chamber of our private lives, we need not obey any rules, conform to any standards, or please anybody—even our preferred self-concepts.

It makes sense, then, that dreams would be more revered by disenfranchised groups—women, African Americans, indigenous peoples, and the less educated, for example—who have often been denied other sources of power. Turning within for guidance in a treacherous world, experienced dreamers find hidden intelligence in the chaotic tangle of what appears when consciousness slips. As a means of direct revelation, dreaming is inherently subversive, often threatening the established order, be it political or personal. For this reason, dreams are often demonized or belittled in hierarchical societies and honored in more egalitarian ones. In some societies, the art of cultivating and interpreting dreams has become a cultural expertise and a veritable means of survival. As one Zinacantec Mayan shaman explained: "We dream to save our lives."[11]

When Harriet Tubman, the leader of the Underground Railroad, led hundreds of slaves to freedom with nothing but the clothes she wore and a pistol, she relied heavily upon her dreams for guidance.[12] She told her biographer, Sarah Bradford, that she often dreamed of flying "like a bird" over the towns, fields, and mountains ahead, when she was guiding fugitives north. Whenever she saw danger in her dreams, Tubman changed their route the next day. After one such dream, she avoided a posse by having her group cross a nearby river, removing their scent from the trail. Tubman made thirteen expeditions altogether, and she never lost a passenger.

Three decades later, a woman who came to be known as Madam C. J. Walker had a dream of her own.[13] The daughter of freed slaves who died when she was young, Sarah survived abuse at the hands of her sister's husband, and the murder of her husband by a white lynch mob, to move to St. Louis where she worked as a cook and housecleaner. When her hair started falling out from stress, Sarah had a dream in which a black man gave her the formula for an ointment she could rub in her scalp to help her hair grow back. It worked, and Sarah started a business selling hair products to black women. It took off like wildfire. Traveling throughout the Americas and the Caribbean to market her goods, Sarah provided jobs for over one thousand saleswomen, and in nine short years, she became the first female self-made millionaire.

A century later, Liberian peace activist Leymah Gbowee followed a dream to lead a mass women's movement to end the war in their country.[14] Gbowee was a survivor of domestic abuse and the mother of four who worked with ex–child soldiers when she dreamed that God told her to "gather the women and pray for peace." She did not feel qualified for the job and tried to find someone else to do it. But when fellow workers convinced her that the "dream bearer is the dream carrier," Gbowee began passing out flyers in markets, mosques, and churches that read: "We are tired! We are tired of our children being killed! We are tired of being raped! Women, wake up—you have a voice in the peace process!" In a few short years, she led thousands of Muslim and Christian women in a nonviolent protest against the war, threatening sex strikes and public disrobing until peace was declared in 2003.

Dreams can also erupt as a disturbing, unsettling force. In early April 1865, President Lincoln had a dream that left him, in his words, "strangely annoyed." The White House was filled with sobbing mourners in his dream, and there was a "corpse wrapped in funeral vestments" in the East Room; when Lincoln asked who it was, he was told it was "the President. He was killed by an assassin!"[15] The president kept this dream to himself for a couple of weeks before telling his wife, bodyguard, and a few friends. They tried to reassure him by saying that the dream probably meant nothing. A few days after their conversation, Lincoln was assassinated.

Tubman, Walker, Gbowee, and Lincoln were exceptional dreamers. Their dreams (at least the ones that made it into historical records) had a clarity and foreknowledge that is rare among the infinitely various visions that come in the night to receptive sleepers. Most of our dreams are of another order, for the realm of conscious sleep experience is an astonishingly wide one, a veritable bestiary of real and imagined creatures.

The Diversity of Dreams

I was surprised to discover that the word *dream* is simply defined as a "series of thoughts, images, or emotions occurring during sleep."[16] In other words, it refers to everything we experience asleep. The definition does not clarify whether the experiences are perceptions or inventions, coming from outside or inside the dreamer. And rightly so. The need to make these distinctions, to bifurcate experience into opposing dualities, is a uniquely Western one that is unfamiliar to most of the world's cultures.

Surveys of oral and written dream narratives from around the world and throughout history indicate that most peoples describe a wide variety of experiences under the heading of dreams, regardless of their natures or origins.[17] Artemidorus, who wrote the earliest known guide to dream interpretation in the second century AD after consulting with hundreds of dreamers and "much-despised diviners of the marketplace" throughout the Middle East, identified five types of dreams: dreams that hide truth beneath figures, visions we perceive awake or asleep, oracles delivered by angels and saints, fantasies that fulfill our waking desires, and apparitions that frighten "weak infants and ancient men."[18]

Five hundred years earlier on the subcontinent of India, the wandering scholar and father of Ayurvedic medicine, Charaka, classified dreams this way: those that reflect what was seen, heard, or experienced in waking life; those that foretell the future; those that reflect a disturbance in the body; those that dramatize fantasies; and those that gratify desires.[19] Two millennia later on the North American continent, Edgar Cayce named four remarkably similar categories: physical, psychological, precognitive, and spiritual.[20] Clearly, dreams do not constitute a single species; they are many.

Not only are there many kinds of dreams, but there are as many dreamers as there are sentient beings on the planet, and each of us dreams after his or her own fashion, as novelist Thomas Mann once noted.[21] I didn't realize how true his words were until I had a curious experience with my friend Barbara, a psychiatric nurse turned Jungian counselor, years ago. We were visiting in her office one day when a gust of wind blew open the window over her desk and swept piles of typewritten pages into the air. They swooped, fluttered, twisted, and twirled like falling leaves, and when we gathered them up, I realized they were her clients' dreams.

"How in the world are you going to figure out which dreams belong to which clients?" I asked, handing over a handful of sheets.

"It's easy," she answered, sorting papers into files. "Dreams can't help but reveal the identities of their dreamers. They're like fingerprints."

I felt the fool for my surprise at her answer, having never imagined that dreams bear the signatures of their owners. I must have thought they were universal and indistinguishable as snowflakes or pollen, whose differences emerge only upon microscopic examination. Obviously, I had not spent the hours studying dreams the way Barbara had, to see through the veil of their common themes to the sure signs of authorship.

Dreaming occurs in a unique context, when our brains are highly stimulated but we are cut off from the sensory input and waking inhibitions that ordinarily stabilize our perceptions. As a result, our brains and minds display a remarkable fluidity amidst the varied individual terrains of our psyches. They move like schools of tiny fish, darting here and there, parting ways and reuniting, in endlessly changing configurations, like the chaotic self-organizing systems they appear to be. At present, several lines of evidence support the notion that our dreaming brains operate on the edge of chaos, albeit a self-organizing one that responds with enormous sensitivity to subtle influences, not unlike the weather systems that bedevil forecasters.[22] Our subconsciously held beliefs are like the rocks and riverbanks that shape those currents, our dreams the tracings. I suspect we have only begun to identify the myriad subtle influences that instigate the flow.

By nature subjective, ephemeral, and mercurial, dreams defy capture. Try to grab one whole from your sleep, like a fish from water, and it will it squirm, flash, and stream through your fingers. The very process of remembering and recounting dreams translates them into the foreign language of our waking lives and social worlds, and we probably use our imaginations to fill in the blanks without even realizing it. As the great Latin American writer Jorge Luis Borges observed: "If we think of the dream as a work of fiction—and I think it is—it may be that we continue to spin tales when we wake and later when we recount them."[23] Interpretation can further twist and mangle these wild creatures. No wonder people throughout history have found dreams to be true and false, guiding and misleading, clear and confusing, personal and collective, real and symbolic, meaningless and revelatory, imagined from within and received from without, about the past, the present, and the future, of this world and of many others.

Despite the plethora of dream types and styles, researcher Kelly Bulkeley points out that most people make a fundamental distinction between everyday dreams rooted in the experiences of our ordinary, waking lives and those occasional, extraordinary dreams that seem to come from powers beyond our personal existences.[24] In the Homeric lore of sixth century BC Greece, what were considered true dreams were sent by the gods through the Gate of Horn, and ordinary, unreliable ones were caused by physiological and emotional disturbances that came through the Gate of Ivory. Centuries later, Carl Jung made a similar distinction between big and little dreams after visiting the Pueblo Indians of North America and the Elgoni peoples of East Africa, both known for their cultural expertise in dreaming.[25] Even Descartes, who considered dreams to be the very models of unreliable knowledge, acknowledged that some rare ones offer glimpses of genuine truth.

While big dreams are clearly a species apart from ordinary ones, the everyday ones filled with the detritus of our days can also take us outside of ourselves, reflecting the communities we inhabit back at us as much as our inner workings do.

13

ORDINARY DREAMS: WHEN ONE HAND WASHES THE OTHER

The writer William Golding once observed that "sleep is when all the unsorted stuff comes flying out as from a dustbin upset in a high wind."[1] Dream researchers report that most of that "unsorted stuff" is a reiteration of common waking life experiences, just a little jumbled up. As the Roman poet Claudian observed in the first century, "hunters dream of woods and beasts, judges of cases, and runners of races." I know an accountant who frequently dreams of adding up long columns of figures in search of the elusive zero. I often find myself walking along lakeshores looking for agates—a favorite hobby of mine—in my dreams. Islamic dream texts called these garden-variety dreams *azgha*, which translates as a "handful of dried grass and weeds."[2] Penelope, in Homer's *Odyssey*, called them cobwebs. Writer Stephen King even referred to them as a kind of "mental or spiritual flatulence."[3] They do seem to display a digestive process at work, breaking down our daily lives into fragments that are mixed, remixed, and gradually disintegrated. It is a process that does not require our conscious involvement and appears to proceed happily without it. As Carl Jung explained:

"The dream itself wants nothing: it is a self-evident content, a plain natural fact like the sugar in the blood of a diabetic or the fever in a patient with typhus."[4] These dreams rarely call our attention and usually dissipate upon waking, sinking back into the unconsciousness from whence they came.

I admit, if I have a dream that I'm running late for class, eating handfuls of chocolate chip cookies, or writing a poem in another language, I usually do not bother to write it down, even though seemingly insignificant dreams have given me great insights in the past. I also tend to discard dreams that seem too jumbled, ludicrous, or boring. The moment I decide a dream is unimportant from my waking perspective, I just cannot motivate myself to do the work of dredging it up, putting it into words, and writing it down. That split-second judgment, which Sigmund Freud aptly called a form of censorship, sends these dreams scurrying like cockroaches from light. For better or for worse, dreams often escape our awareness.

The tendency for dreams to dissipate upon waking is often considered to be a protective device. Freud claimed it protected our egos, our preferred self-images, from the self-knowledge our nightly adventures provide. It could just as easily protect our dreams from the distortions of memory and interpretation, the ways of the waking world. Dream recall involves a two-way relationship between the dreamer and the dreamed in which both parties must be willing. That relationship breaks down, or simply does not come into play, when seemingly ordinary dreams occur. Despite their routine repeated disappearances, ordinary dreams may still perform the invisible labors of sleep: remembering and recovering. I have a friend whose father walked out on her family one morning without explanation when she was ten years old. In the years that followed, she dreamed of his leaving many times, each time in a different way: taking the exit ramp off the highway, following a runaway kite, dashing for a phone call in another city, bringing the Christmas tree to another house, and so on. They were familiar, straightforward dreams that did not require interpretation. Something in her just could not get what had happened and continued to chew on it like an old bone, trying to digest the unacceptable.

Fortunately, my friend's dreams did not return her to the site and repeat the trauma. Instead, they continually reformulated the event, portraying it as a mistaken judgment in one, a reaching for something else in another, and a function of getting hopelessly lost in another, all of which shifted her interpretation of his actions ever so slightly and defused the intensity of her responses. Rosalind Cartwright, who conducts research on dream series like this one, has observed that a "progressive down-scaling of disturbing emotion" occurs through dreaming over the course of a single night, not to mention months and years.[5] In retrospect, it seems that my friend's dreams facilitated her reconciliation with the event that tore her family apart as a child, but they may simply have revealed its progression. At any rate, the dreams stopped happening.

Almost every known system of dream categorization has a place for what could be called psychological dreams like the ones my friend had. They are often attributed to some kind of physical or psychological disturbance within the dreamer, which may explain why dream sharing has played a central role in healing practices around the world, including in Western psychotherapy. Dreams have a way of dramatizing whatever is agitating the dreamer, what could be called the karmic traces—to use a term from Hindu and Buddhist philosophy—currently at play in one's life.[6] Some researchers propose that dreams begin with the kernel of an emotion and spin a story to justify it, like dressing to suit one's mood. But dreams are rarely so obvious as the ones reported by my friend. As Artemidorus observed centuries ago, many dreams that "hide beneath figures" and cannot be taken at face value; they require telling and consideration to relate them to our lives—if they do, in fact, have any relation to our lives.

I once had a dream in which I was happily holding hands with a woman I felt very close to, only to realize that razor blades were hidden in her palm and were cutting me to shreds. When I woke up, I jumped out of bed and ran to make sure all the windows and doors in my apartment were locked. As the day progressed, I kept asking myself, feverishly: "Who is it? Who is pretending to be my friend while hurting me? Who shouldn't I trust?" I looked askance at everyone who crossed my path that day, and my paranoia grew by the hour. Then, when I was berating myself later that night over some mistake I had made, it occurred to me in a streak of sudden comprehension: I was my own worst friend, hiding beneath the figure of the cutting woman.

After years of working with dreams in a variety of styles and contexts, I have come to the conclusion that befuddling dreams are meant to do just that: confuse, disturb, and challenge our waking points of view. The very act of remembering a dream shuffles together the cards of our waking and sleeping thought, subtly decentering and altering each. Something like a chemical reaction can occur when nocturnal and diurnal realities mingle. When I had the dream of holding hands with razor blades, the image and feeling of it stayed with me all day until a meaning suddenly fell into place with that shocking insight. It is as if the act of superimposing my night and day lives created an eruption that sliced like lightning through both worlds and united them as one, at least for a moment, etching the visceral depiction of the ways I hurt myself into my mind forever. I cannot say that I have never criticized myself since, but when I do, and the dream comes to mind, I let go of that hand like a hot potato.

The Personal and Communal Roots of Dreams

Ever since Aristotle declared that dreams come from within the self in the fourth century BC, Westerners have found reflections of themselves and their predicaments in their dreams. "I've always used dreams the way you'd use mirrors to look at something you couldn't see head-on, the way that you use a mirror to look at your hair in the back," explained Stephen King.[7] "To me that's what dreams are supposed to do." The prefrontal cortex—the part of our brains that assesses situations, applies moral values, and then imagines consequences—is deactivated when we sleep; as a result, we do not temper our impulses in our dreams. Secrets (even those we keep from ourselves) have a way of slipping out.

Until the advent of scientific medicine, physicians and folk healers relied upon their patients' dreams for additional information in making diagnoses the way doctors now use tests. Hippocrates, known as the father of Western medicine, and his counterparts in ancient India and China routinely asked their patients to report their dreams in the belief that the soul perceives the causes of illness during sleep and produces images reflecting those invisible conditions. The Roman physician Galen, later explained: "It is likely that in sleep the soul, having gone into the depths of the body and retreated from the external perceptions, perceives the dispositions throughout the body and forms an impression… as though these things were already present." Galen seems to be alluding to an unconscious sensibility or intelligence that can access knowledge not consciously available to us. It could be based in what biologists now term our interoceptive senses, which receive information from within our bodies, such as the sensation of being hungry, thirsty, or aroused—or the position of your body or when you need to use the bathroom.

Neurologist Oliver Sacks noted that his patients sometimes dream of their disorders before their onset.[8] One woman had a string of terrifying dreams: of being imprisoned in a castle the shape of her body, of being enchanted and bewitched, of becoming a stone statue, of falling into a sleep so deep she could not be roused. The next morning, her family could not wake her, for she had become catatonic overnight. Another patient began to dream of moving in slow motion, of being frozen in place, or of rushing so fast he couldn't stop, with time and space "switching scales," before he developed Parkinson's disease. "One must assume in such cases," Sacks wrote, "that the disease was already affecting neural function, and that the unconscious mind, the dreaming mind, was more sensitive to this than the waking mind."

My friend Barbara, the psychiatric nurse who became a Jungian therapist, was renowned for her ability to detect early signs of disease in the images of her clients' dreams. She once sent a client to a dermatologist for a full body exam on the basis of a dream without seeing any concerning spots. The doctor found, and successfully treated, a dangerous melanoma. Barbara herself survived two life-threatening cancers, and when she called to tell me she had dreamed the third one would kill her, I knew she was probably right—as much as I fought the verdict.

This sense of a hidden interior from which dreams emerge was revived in the West with the discovery of the unconscious, first identified by the Renaissance physician Paracelsus and later made famous by the work of Sigmund Freud. Carl Jung expanded upon Freud's notion of a personal unconscious to propose the existence of a collective unconscious, a repository of ancestral experience we share as human beings.[9] In so doing, he opened the door to the possibility that our dreams could refer to what is brewing collectively, beyond the confines of our individual lives. Thomas Mann implied such a possibility when he wrote in *The*

Magic Mountain: "Now I know that it is not out of our single souls we dream. We dream anonymously and communally, if each after his fashion. The great soul of which we are a part may dream through us, in our manner of dreaming, its own secret dreams."[10]

For many non-Western tribal peoples, dreams not only reflect individual conditions, but they also reveal what is occurring and unfolding in the larger world. In this understanding, the dreaming self—called the breath soul, the free soul, or the eye soul in various traditions and resembling something akin to one's reflection in a mirror or shadow on the ground—visits with the spirits of surrounding animals, plants, landforms, ancestors, and holy ones.[11] As anthropologist Vincent Crapanzano explained: "Much of what we in the West call psychological and locate in some sort of internal space ('in the head,' 'in the mind,' 'in the brain,' 'in consciousness,' 'in the psyche') is understood in many cultures in manifestly nonpsychological terms and located in other 'spaces.'"[12] Dreaming is a form of communication and exchange with others, something that certain dreamers (usually leaders, healers, or artists) undertake to mediate tensions, gain understanding, and retrieve knowledge. That knowledge can take the form of a beadwork design, a ritual song, a ceremonial dance, or the healing properties of an herb, and it's often shared for the good of the community.

From a tribal perspective, those raised and educated within a Western worldview tend to privatize dreams, regarding them as individual property rather than communal resources.[13] We assume authorship of our dreams as if we were immune to, and untouched by, outside influences. However, that is a relatively recent notion, even in the West, and it appears to have arisen alongside the practice of solitary sleep. Before the Enlightenment, when communal sleep was prevalent, people considered themselves to be permeable, loose collections of separable selves vulnerable to outside influences, able to be swayed, sundered and possessed, for better or for worse. Our language retains axioms that reflect this understanding; we speak of cracking up, breaking down, being overwhelmed and succumbing to illness or despair. The word *individual* didn't come into use in the West until the seventeenth century with the advent of merchant capitalism and imperialism. It literally means "indivisible," unable to be divided but also connotes independence, uniqueness, and self-possession.

This sense of separateness from the surrounding world is foreign to many traditions where personhood is more fluid and interwoven with the people, animals, and features of the environment. It is also increasingly contradicted by recent scientific discoveries in a variety of fields. In the neurosciences, for example, the revelation that our brains develop throughout life, translating our encounters with our environments into the circuitry of our brain-based knowledge, suggests that the world lives in us as much as we live in it.[14] The universe we experience through our perceptual filters is inscribed into our brains and tattooed onto our imaginations, shaping our experiences by day and by night. If our dreams are the unbridled expressions of our imaginations, as some neuroscientists argue, the random firings of our neural circuits, as others suggest, or a second cognitive system, as still others propose, we must remember that our brains, minds, and imaginations are constructed by the worlds in which we live.

To some extent, the difference lies in the attitudes we hold toward our sleep experiences, for dreaming is both an innate capacity and a cultivated art. Dreamers have often noted that the more attention they give to their dreams, the more they remember, and the more valuable they become. I have heard the practice likened to developing a relationship with a wild animal or young child, requiring patience, respect, and responsiveness before each opens to the other. This may be the reason so many peoples make offerings and prayers before asking for, or discussing, a dream. It is a way of placing themselves into the respectful posture capable of receiving and honoring what is given.

One Hand Washes the Other

Ulu Temay, a Huichol shaman, explained: "If a person doesn't believe in his dreams, he might say, 'It's only a dream; it's not real; the gods aren't really taking to me.' Little by little, everything will become less clear… If one doesn't do what a dream has directed… one won't be able to dream well anymore."[15] Edgar Cayce expressed a similar understanding when he observed that dreams instruct or deceive, guide or confuse, depending upon our attitudes, motivations, and past responses.[16]

There is a relationship between the dreamer and his or her dreams, regardless of whether the encompassing culture supports or discourages it. Temay and Cayce appear to suggest that one's actions influence the quality of one's dreams. The renowned sixteenth-century Cabalist Isaac Luria expressed a similar sentiment when he wrote that the divine figures, or "answering angels," who appear in dreams spring from the actions of the dreamer.[17] Some tell the truth, explained Luria, and others tell lies, depending on what the dreaming host does by day with the information given by night. For this reason, many indigenous peoples show their children how to cultivate an honest and healthy relationship with their dreams. French anthropologist Florence Brunois reported that the Kasua people of Papua New Guinea encourage young people to observe animals in the wild, pick one to focus upon, dream of being that animal, and slowly incorporate its most salient characteristics, creating a kinship so strong, they were forbidden to hunt that animal again.[18] Under Kasua tutelage, dreaming becomes a means of communing with the nonhuman universe; of learning about, and empathizing with, a larger community that does not necessarily place humans at the center.

I occasionally dream that I am someone else of another age, sex, or circumstance. I have been an aged trader in Turkey, a young woman in the time of Jesus, a deaf-mute tied to a tree, a mother who has lost her child—even a bear coming out of hibernation. Sometimes I dream someone else's life story as if I were watching a movie. When I wake up, I often feel slightly altered, as if the streams of experience I dreamed were actually my own. My sense of self becomes a little more open and elastic, and I feel affinities with people, animals, countries, and situations I never really had before. The next day I might look for the plant with the pointed leaves I saw in my dream or visit with the neighbor whose daughter died in a car accident with more ease. I treasure these dreams because they enlarge my empathy and lend me a host of experiences I could not get any other way.

In a sense, we get what we ask for—or find what we are looking for—in our dreams. If we want to understand ourselves more fully, our dreams hold up mirrors. If we want to know the creatures around us better, they come to us in our dreams. If we want to make peace with the ancestors, our dreams tell us what to do. A hospice nurse once told me that people die the way they live; I suspect the same is true of the way we dream. We dream the way we live.

Artemidorus, the man who interviewed thousands of dreamers in Eastern and Western rural and urban cultures throughout the Middle East during the second century AD, struggled to define the nature of dreams. In the end, he decided not to take sides in the debate over whether "our dreaming comes to us externally from the gods or whether there is some internal cause which disposes the soul in a certain way and causes a natural event to happen to it."[19] However, in his phrasing of the debate, Artemidorus hinted at a third possibility: that there exists a reflexive, reciprocating relationship between what we perceive as inside and outside, subject and object, human and divine. Think of it this way: when one hand washes the other, each is actor and acted upon. So it is, Artemidorus seems to suggest, with the dream and the dreamer. Each impacts and evokes the other. As Ralph Waldo Emerson cryptically observed, "My dreams are not me; they are not Nature, or the Not-me; they are both. They have a double consciousness, at one sub- and objective."

My head spins when I try to grasp this concept. I understand it best when I think of dreams I have had involving family members. I know that my relatives are not literally walking through my night world, but I have not made them up out of the blue either. A lifetime of interactions has created and refined their appearances in my dreams. They act like themselves and so do I; we cannot help it. If one of us breaks out of character, my daytime relationship with that person changes a little, even if I do not want it to, which may explain why some cultures ask dreamers to apologize to people they have wronged in their dreams. The older I get, the more I realize that my relationships continue to evolve through waking and dreaming interactions, even after someone dies. It is an ongoing process of discovery with no dotted line dividing what is out there from what is in here. American psychologist James Hillman described it well:

> Perhaps there is a work going on in the dreams a prolonged cooking of obdurate residues that dissolve the all-too-solid flesh of remembered persons into… shades of themselves, so that they may depart, freed of their attachments, and we may live in their presence without being oppressed by their life.[20]

Dream Visitations and Travels

While cultures across the globe describe the kinds of sleep and the varieties of dreams in remarkably similar ways, our understandings of what happens when we dream could not be more different. Ethnological research indicates that people in a vast array of societies around the world consider dreams to be a form of soul travel.[21] Abolitionist Harriet Tubman told her biographer, Sarah Bradford, that her spirit left her body when she fell asleep and visited "other scenes and places, not only in this world, but in the world of spirits." A member of the Kalapalo Indian tribe of Central Brazil told anthropologist Ellen Basso: "When we are asleep, we are sound asleep, and our akũa [which Basso translated as "interactive selves"] wake up and begin to roam around. Then we dream."[22] The notion that each of us has an immaterial soul, a shadow or secret self, which separates from the body in sleep, is ubiquitous among non-Westernized peoples.

Educated Westerners usually dismiss this idea as superstition, however. Bradford seemed to doubt Harriet Tubman's report of her dream life when she wrote that she "imagined" her spirit left her body in sleep. Some scientists and philosophers propose that the thoughts and feelings we ascribe to the soul result from random firings of nerve cells in the brain stem, something like the foam and flotsam from crashing waves. In their view, dreams are indelibly tied to the physical body. It is the age-old conflict between spiritualists and materialists, and I have come to suspect that both have a piece of the truth. When it comes to understanding sleep, we are like the proverbial blind men describing an elephant, as researcher Robert Stickgold often says.[23] Each of us has an angle on what transpires, but none of us has the whole picture.

One of the most commonly described features of dreaming is the sense of hurried movement. It seems we are always jumping, falling, flying, running, or driving in our dreams, and if we finally come to a standstill, we usually wake up. We repeatedly encounter novel, confusing, and disturbing situations, get lost and run late, forever trying to get ourselves properly oriented in time and space. Scientists explain that the cells in the brain stem that register subtle changes in balance when we move are more stimulated when we are asleep than when we are awake, so it is no wonder we feel like we are undertaking epic odysseys in our dreams, even though our bodies remain relatively still.[24] But the fundamental question remains: do neuronal firings in our brains create the sense of hurried movement in our dreams, or do our dream travels stimulate the neuronal firing? All we know for sure is that they occur simultaneously.

Encounters with the dead in dreams or visitations like the one described at the beginning of this chapter have been reported in virtually all cultures and times. They lend themselves to the idea that some immaterial aspect of ourselves can leave our bodies and reach across space and time. Experiences of sleep paralysis, when we wake but cannot move, contribute to the sense that some part of us can exist outside our bodies. Some psychologists, and even a few neuroscientists, have called this part of us the witnessing or observing self, noting it emerges in dreams, meditations, and other reflective states. All of these common human experiences support to the notion of dream travel, regardless of whether one believes that we possess souls capable of separating from our bodies.

Dream reports of journeying to other places and discovering things that turn out to be there in waking life press the issue of travel even further. Ancient Buddhist practitioners, and even a few contemporary lamas, have reportedly found buried treasures after visiting the locations in their dreams.[25] I once had a dream in which I saw a white van roll over into a stream where white lilies sprung up, only to learn the next day that two friends in another part of the country had turned over in their white van, landing upside down in a shallow river. One of them had died and been resuscitated.

Hans Berger, the man who invented the EEG that enabled scientists to explore what happens when we sleep, had a similar experience.[26] One morning, while out horseback riding, Berger was accidentally thrown into the path of a fast-approaching horse-driven artillery cannon. He expected to be crushed instantly, but miraculously, the cannon's driver was able to stop. That evening Berger received a telegram from his sister posted shortly after his near accident, expressing her urgent concern for his welfare because she had just had a terrible ominous feeling about him.

These could be coincidences, noted and remembered because of their rarity and seeming impossibility. Maybe my dreaming self and Berger's sister's conscious awareness somehow transported themselves to the site of the events. Maybe these death-defying incidents projected themselves over to us, catching us in receptive moments. Perhaps we all met in some middle ground where time and space collide. There are realms of experience that defy conceptualization, much as people like me try to pin them down. Regardless of how we understand them, incidents like these can change people's lives. Berger switched his career from astronomy to medicine after his encounter in order to investigate what he called psychic energy. As a result, we know much more about what happens when we sleep, dream, and awaken.

Ultimately, the question is not whether we dream inside or outside of ourselves but where dreaming occurs that it manages to include both. Sufi philosophers historically maintained that dreams occur in a "third world" of imagination situated alongside the physical, where meanings embodied as images have a nearly autonomous existence.[27] The fifth century philosopher and Christian bishop Synesius considered this third world to be something like a halfway house "between spirit and matter, which makes communication between the two possible."[28] In the Hindu cosmology of the *Brhadāranyaka Upanishad*, dreaming takes place in the "twilight juncture" between the tangible world and an intangible one beyond, neither of which is fully real or unreal. Other peoples describe a shadow world, an intermediate state, a spiritual plane, or a mythic realm where souls travel and all of time and space intersect. Some explain that we do not have dreams inside of us; rather, we live inside our dreams while sleeping.

Whatever words and concepts are used to describe it, the realms we traverse in our dreams are commonly thought to coincide and intersect with the worlds we experience by day. Whether personal or communal, they take us outside ourselves, pointing forward, backward, and into worlds far beyond the known.

14

BIG DREAMS: MYSTERIOUS ENCOUNTERS IN SLUMBER

English novelist Emily Brontë once wrote: "I've dreamt in my life dreams that have stayed with me ever after, and changed my ideas; they've gone through and through me, like wine through water, and altered the color of my mind." Big dreams—the ones that stand out, startle, and strike us, leave their mark and refuse to be forgotten—are recognized as significant life experiences in most non-Western cultures and by many in Western cultures as well. They go by a variety of names: lucky dreams, holy dreams, titanic dreams, archetypal dreams, clear dream visions, and dreams under the influence of a deity.[1]

Pioneering sleep researcher and psychiatrist William Dement described one such dream, an "exceptionally vivid and realistic" one he had early in his career:

> I had inoperable cancer of the lung. I remember as though it were yesterday looking at the ominous shadow in my chest X-ray and realizing that the entire right lung was infiltrated. I experienced the incredible anguish of knowing my life

> was soon to end, that I would never see my children grow up, and that none of this would have happened if I had quit cigarettes when I first learned of their carcinogenic potential. I will never forget the surprise, joy, and exquisite relief of waking up.[2]

Dement noted that this dream was unlike others he had had. It lacked the daily residues, the sudden dislocations, and confusing transmutations that typically characterize ordinary dreams, the qualities that make it easy to suppose that dreams result from spontaneous, random firings in our brains. It was utterly clear, direct, and undeniable, a warning he could not ignore. Dement stopped smoking that day.

Dreams That Matter

Big dreams appear to be of another order altogether. They have a remarkable clarity and a profound sense of portent that alter and inform us for life. They are not just remixes of memory traces from past experiences or imagined possibilities; they seem to create new experiences beyond the range of what we have known. It is as if they dropped in from a greater, more encompassing reality. They are, to use a phrase from anthropologist Amira Mittermaier, "dreams that matter," ones that address the dreamer and call for a response in waking life.[3] Mittermaier notes that, according to Islamic tradition, dreams like these "allow the future to fold into the present." In short, they may be revelatory.

Many occur in childhood, before our socialized selves take over and colonize our inner lives. Writer Anne Rice had a momentous dream as a very young girl, in which a woman made of marble was walking down the street and a voice told her the figure was her grandmother.[4] It may not seem like much, but Rice later explained: "When a dream is that intense, when it is that otherworldly, it's a little frightening. It's almost as if you saw into another realm. You saw something that had to do with heritage or lineage that went beyond what you could see with rational eyes." Rice related that she has had a lifelong fear and horror of the pure idea, the "thing that is detached from the flesh" like the marble woman. The entire thrust of her work has been to say, in her words: "Listen to the lessons of the flesh."

In retrospect, it appears that Rice's childhood vision set the tone and direction for her life, but that may only seem so in hindsight. In the end, it does not really matter whether the dream guided the life or the life found the dream; it is the ongoing dialogue between our dreaming and waking lives that matters. As a Muslim dream interpreter in Cairo told Mittermaier, "The waking state gives to the dream and the dream gives, in turn, to the awakened state."[5]

The most common and widespread example of a big dream is a visit from someone who has died. People often dream of the deceased as if they were still alive and they are playing cards, making dinner, or doing whatever they used to do together, but there are other rare occasions when the dead seemingly present themselves with something to communicate. The sense of certainty that accompanies these encounters—in our waking or dreaming lives—is hard to grasp. I have heard people describe these visits as more real than real life, which is a sensation I have come to both trust and suspect.

Even though neuroscientists have demonstrated our capacity to create phantoms we experience as real, as in phantom limbs that itch or burn, that knowledge rarely diminishes the impact of a visit from a loved one who has died. Nor does the discovery that spiritual experiences like this, which are drenched with emotion, often coincide with activation of the temporal lobes of our brains. The feelings that accompany these meetings are stronger than any ideas we may hold about what is real and what is not. For this reason, visits from the dead have swung open the door to a spiritual life for people the world over, and their stories can be found in the holy books of almost every religion. Dreaming may be the biological basis for spirituality.

Many months after my high school friend Patsy killed herself, I dreamed that she ran up to me, thrust a bunch of letters into my hand to mail, and dashed off before I could say anything. When I dropped the envelopes into the mail slot, I noticed the last one was addressed to "The World." It was a short, simple, remarkably realistic dream. I knew Patsy was dead in the dream, and she apparently did too, because she gave me her final messages. Patsy acted like herself, someone who usually found the tasks of daily life to be overwhelming and often leaned on me to do things like this for her. When I woke from the dream, I felt what I had often experienced around Patsy when she was alive, a mixture of affection and annoyance with a touch of awe. But when I realized that she had asked me to deliver her message to the world, I felt honored—and surprisingly invigorated. The dream exchange melted the survivor's guilt that had oppressed me since her suicide into a sense of purpose. I would keep her memory alive and would work on behalf of the Patsys of our world, the misunderstood and mistreated among us. In a sense, the dream returned me to the world and to that web of obligations and exchanges that constitute community.

Dream encounters with the dead often involve an exchange of some sort. Messages are relayed, requests made, warnings and reassurances given. Carl Jung reported that his dead father asked him for marital advice in a dream, as he wanted to prepare for his wife's arrival, which Jung took as news that his mother would die soon. The appearance of the dead in our dreams can prepare us for changes to come or compel us to do what needs to be done. They bring us back into relationship after loss has occurred, erode the isolation and self-centeredness of grief, and make us remember that we belong, forever interconnected and interdependent.

Visions and Visitations

Nearly thirty years ago, when I first moved to the small town where I now live, I found a car mechanic who worked out of his home garage to give my Datsun a tune-up. The place was filled with cars in various stages of repair. He told me to come back on Monday, but when I did, the garage was empty, except for a wooden easel, where my mechanic stood painting. When I asked what was going on, he told me that he had gone to the mountains for wood the day before, taken a small nap under a pine tree, and when he woke and opened his eyes, "Our Lady" (of Guadalupe) appeared before him. "I've been painting ever since," he explained, "trying to get all the details right before I forget." Turning back to the easel, he added, "I'll have your car for you on Wednesday."

It is a short step from meeting a deceased loved one in a dream to encountering a spiritual guide. In the eleventh century, a Japanese woman known as Lady Sarashina recorded the following dream she had had long before, one that carried her through years of suffering:

> Amida Buddha was standing in the far end of our garden. I could not see him clearly, for a layer of mist seemed to separate us, but when I peered through the mist… He glowed with a golden light, and one of his hands was stretched out… He had said, "I shall leave now, but later

I shall return to fetch you.[6]

The message was cohesive, direct, and authoritative, as is often the case in big dreams like this. The voice, which a friend of mine humorously calls the intercom voice, is indisputable. As the Persian Sufi poet Rumi declared: "Everyone understands this voice when it comes. It speaks with the same authority to Turk and Kurd, Persian Arab, Ethiopian, one language!"

Around the world and millennia later, a rural Michigan woman told psychologist Edward Hoffman a remarkably similar dream she'd had at the age of four.[7] She was walking up a hill through tall pines at sunset. When she got to the top, she saw a "large, bright, white, transparent figure" coming toward her until he stood right next to her. The figure took her hand and said: "Don't be afraid. I'll always be with you."

I have yet to find a religious tradition whose texts do not include dream narratives, be it the story of Jacob's ladder, Mohammed's night journey, Vishnu's world, or Queen Maya's magnificent white elephant. Dreams supply a good part of humanity's knowledge of the greater whole, whether it's understood to be God, the Tao, chance, or something else.

A friend once asked me why Buddhists dream of Bodhisattvas and Catholics dream of Jesus and Mother Mary. Even though I have known people to dream of deities from traditions of which they have no knowledge, the point is well taken. We clothe our divinities—both the angels and the demons—with our own beliefs, conscious and unconscious That may be the only way our brains can perceive the energy passing in that moment. Perhaps, our beliefs actually create our images of the divine and our dreaming brains supply the emotional charge that makes them so powerful. Even so, something beyond our beliefs seems to swoop in and inhabit these forms in big dreams because they challenge, comfort, instruct, and move us beyond our previous limitations, for better or for worse.

Dream researcher Kelly Bulkeley has observed that the divine beings who appear in dreams tend to be relatively close to the human realm.[8] They are typically the angels, messengers, and mediators, not the great transcendent Creator gods of the world's religions. That is a good thing, I suspect, because it gives us a little room to consider the advice we are given before acting upon it. After all, "God" has told people to do some terrible things in the past, violating every moral code imaginable. That intercom voice can have many origins.

Fortunately, our lives as mammalian creatures require us to slip in and out of waking and dreaming worlds on a daily basis, fostering a continual dialogue between the two, not domination of one over the other. In this way, we learn to test and assess the voices of our waking and dreaming selves. It is the conversation between sleeping and waking realities, and the small adaptations they induce, that makes us the conscious, forever learning beings that we are.

Prophetic Dreams

When I had breast cancer years ago, my surgeon performed what appeared to be a successful lumpectomy to save my breast. A few nights later, I dreamed of listening to an exquisite blues song with this refrain: "You give it all you got, and you lose it anyway." I dutifully wrote down the dream and forgot about it. Later that day, my surgeon called to report that the margins of the lumpectomy were not clean, and I would have to get a mastectomy after all. "Well," I responded, "we gave it all we got," quoting my dream without even remembering it. In fact, I did not discover the dream until

I reviewed my dream journals to write this book. In retrospect, I imagine my response sounded odd to my surgeon's ear, but the words rolled off my lips like an old church hymn.

There is a recurrent notion throughout history and around the world that dreams can predict the future, but most do not. How some dreams can accurately portray an event yet to unfold is a matter of much speculation—and some interesting theories. Medieval Christian theologians claimed that God reveals "future contingents" in dreams.[9] Aristotle, who discounted the notion of god-sent dreams, wrote with a more scientific attitude: "The movements in sleep are often the starting points for the activities of the day, because the thought for the latter is already started on its way in our nocturnal fancies." The fact that I quoted my dream to my surgeon the next day without remembering it seems to confirm Aristotle's insight. That blues song, both its sadness and its refrain, paved the way for my response the next day.

Our brains are continually building internal models of the outside world. When we are waiting for information to reveal which possibility will unfold in the future—in my case, mastectomy or no mastectomy—we naturally imagine what it would be like to go down either path, preparing ourselves for the best and the worst. Carl Jung called this the prospective function of dreams, in which the unconscious brings together various, perceptions, thoughts, memories, and feelings to envision one's future, creating "something like a preliminary exercise or sketch, or a plan roughed out in advance."[10] This futurizing, as a friend of mine calls it, can create needless worry, but it also prepares us for any number of possible futures. In her book *Crisis Dreaming*, Rosalind Cartwright described numerous dreams that anticipated major life events in people's lives, such as childbirth, illness, and death, and concluded that these dreams "enable us to revise our pictures of our present selves and to rehearse our responses to future challenges."[11]

The moment we remember a dream, write it down, or tell it to someone else, we bring it into our day lives, and charge it with meaning and possibility. In a sense, we breathe life into it and make it more real—more likely to come true. If it is a frightening dream, like the one William Dement had of living with lung cancer, we are compelled to take action to prevent it from coming true. If it is a comforting or inspiring dream, we keep it close to our hearts, remember and refer to it frequently, and do our best to live it out in our lives.

In 1938, President Roosevelt had a dream in which he rose from his bed, looked out the window, and witnessed a terrible crash at the airport near Camp Springs, Maryland.[12] Remarkably, Roosevelt immediately told the dream to a group of congressmen and convinced them to appropriate $10 million to replace the airport with a new one, insisting that "it was imperative to prevent any such crash."

Dreams have started and ended wars and have prompted people to adopt children, take up causes, and leave unhappy marriages. Sometimes it seems to me that dreams seek a moral equilibrium, not just in our own lives, but in the world at large. *Liezi*, a Taoist text from the fourth century, recounts an interesting tale about the dreams of a rich man and his servant: The rich man treats his servant terribly, but the servant is content because he dreams every night of having great powers and pleasures. The rich man, on the other hand, is miserable because he dreams of being abused and overworked every night. Finally, the rich man realizes he can put an end to his misery by treating his servant kindly.[13] While the story may be more about fluctuating opposites—a central tenet of Taoism—than dreams, it shows how our dreaming lives can inform our waking lives and reveal our futures. In the land of dreams, we can find our future selves, as a Wintu lullaby illustrates:

Sleep! Sleep!
In the land of dreams
Find your grownup self
Your future family
Sleep! Sleep![14]

However, finding our future selves and manifesting these selves in the waking world are two different tasks. Whereas most dreams come to us involuntarily, we have to work to wake up. Every time we wake, we make that passage across the waters of forgetting and into another world—a daytime world that runs by entirely different rules.

15

WAKING UP IS HARD TO DO: INTERNAL AND SOCIAL TIME

My father used to pop out of bed at the same time every morning with an eagerness for the day that I have always envied. He would march down the hall to the kitchen, flicking on lights as he went, turn on the radio for the morning news—and wake us all up. I took more after my mother, who rarely showed her face before we left the house, and if she did pad out in her bedroom slippers, we knew to give her a wide berth until she had downed her second cup of coffee. Then, and only then, was she capable of civility.

I was so intent upon skipping my father's morning wake-up call that I sometimes got up in the night, tiptoed out of my bedroom, and found a new, secret hiding place in which to finish sleeping unnoticed. I curled up in the hall closet or under my mother's desk in the basement, even in the laundry basket—anywhere my father wouldn't find me and I could surface slowly into the world of the waking.

Years later, my five-year-old stepdaughter decided she wanted to live with her grandfather, so we arranged for her to stay with him for a week. She lasted two days. When she called begging to return, we asked why (undoubtedly hoping for those words of appreciation parents crave), and she howled into the phone: "He pulls the covers off me when I don't get up in the morning!" Her outrage was stunning. It made me wonder whether we had overindulged her morning grumpiness by taking a good hour to wake her and calling several times before turning on the lights in her room. But then, none of us in that household liked a rude awakening.

How We Wake

The very phrase *rude awakening* implies that the process of becoming conscious should be a kind one, a slow easing into awareness, the way dawn comes over us with the slight stirrings of small critters, the call of one bird and then another as the sky lightens and begins to outline nearby buildings, followed by the crown of color in the east and the first brilliant dusting of light upon the uppermost branches of the trees. I have heard it said that the slow accumulation of early-morning light and sound is nature's way of calling our souls back into our bodies. In cultures that discourage sudden awakenings, people call softly, hum, or sing to entice a sleeper to return to the waking world. The popular folk song "Frère Jacques" may have had its origin in this practice:

Are you sleeping, are you sleeping,
Brother John? Brother John?
Morning bells are ringing! Morning bells are ringing!
Ding, dang, dong. Ding, dang, dong.

I like to imagine that our preindustrial ancestors came to waking awareness slowly, stretching, yawning and rolling over, cuddling and cooing with bedmates, as the room itself gradually materialized with the light of day. But most of us do not have that luxury, if it ever existed. There are kids to feed, cars to start, jobs to get to. More often than not, the ring of an alarm clock catapults us from deep slumber toward the waking world, and hopefully, bright lights and caffeinated drinks carry us the rest of the way.

The long history of sounding clocks suggests that people have not had the leisure for kind awakenings for some time.[1] Ever since water clocks were invented some two thousand years ago, people the world over have attached mechanisms to strike gongs at preset hours. Clock towers have called people to prayer and work in cities from Hong Kong to Cairo to Rio de Janeiro, while those who lived in isolated, rural areas relied often upon roosters to rouse them. In the sixteenth and seventeenth centuries, cuckoo clocks became prized fixtures in the homes of the wealthy. By the twentieth century, wind-up, battery-operated, or electrical clocks could be found in almost every kitchen and bedroom. When factories were converted for military production during World War II, broken alarm clocks could not be replaced, and the shortage in American homes created such havoc in workplaces that the federal government allowed clock companies to resume production before all others. By the end of the century, almost every device, from cars to computers to DVD players, included a time-keeping device.

Each and every one of these ubiquitous timepieces serves to drag us out of our own, innate body time into the socially constructed and enforced clock time we share with others. Like magnets in a field of scattered metal filings, they whip us into line.

Body Clocks

As the Earth turns on its axis, its shadow slides across the seas and continents, marking the onset of each day and night. Every creature, from a single cell of sea plankton to the hundred-foot blue whale, undergoes profound and predictable changes as the degrees of light and temperature shift. Plants lift and drop their leaves; open and close their flowers; and undergo phases of respiration, growth, and photosynthesis. Birds sing, feed, mate, and migrate according to the time of day or season. Mammals emerge from hiding to roam and forage, or return home to rest and sleep. Because life evolved on Earth under the conditions of alternating light and darkness, heat and cold, we are wired to make these shifts for the differing purposes of our waking and sleeping lives—even without environmental cues. It is one of the most basic, visceral ways that all of us participate in nature, something we share with every living thing.

In the fourth century BC, a ship captain serving under Alexander the Great noticed that the leaves of the tamarind tree folded up at night. I am sure he was not the first to observe nocturnal changes in plants, but he may have been the first to write about them. More than two millennia later in the eighteenth century, a French scientist named Jean-Jacques d'Ortous de Mairan noticed that these leaf movements continued to occur in total darkness, proving that they were not responding to changes in light. He thought they might be reacting to shifts in temperature or magnetic fields. By the end of the twentieth century, scientists had demonstrated that daily rhythmic changes in plants, animals, humans—and even bacteria—are driven by internal circadian (meaning daily) clocks that can be influenced by external conditions like light but generally run on their own biological time.[2]

In humans, circadian clocks do more than lift or drop leaves. They are responsible for daily fluctuations in blood pressure, body temperature, immunity, hormones, hunger, thirst, and arousal, including our sleep-wake cycles.[3] These biological rhythms, which we experience as internal time, are probably older than sleep, developed over the course of aeons of evolution on our spinning planet. They facilitate physiological and behavioral changes on a roughly twenty-four-hour cycle no matter what is happening outside, whether a cold front moves in or clouds block the light of the sun.

That is why people experience jet lag when traveling across time zones; their internal clocks continue to run in accordance with the place they left behind, not the one to which they have come, and it can take some time to realign the two. The most remarkable thing, at least for me, is that our internal body clocks can be readjusted by environmental cues. We may get jet lag for a few days when we ask our circadian rhythms to adapt to a vastly different schedule of day and night cycles on the other side of the Earth, but they can do it.[4]

Eventually, human circadian cycles adjust to new time zones, primarily by exposure to daylight. The sun is our original timekeeper, after all. Photosensitive ganglion cells in our eyes inform our brains of the general level of light outside, which in turn, time the secretion of melatonin to synchronize internal rhythms with external ones. However, there are circadian clocks throughout our bodies, not just in our brains. Peripheral clocks exist in tissues of the esophagus, lungs, liver, pancreas, spleen, thymus, and skin, and they don't always fall in line with the master clock in the brain. Some appear to adjust at different rates, and this desynchronization can feel strange.[5] The symptoms we typically associate with jet lag, time changes, and shift work—disorientation, headaches, fatigue, insomnia, irritability, depression, and constipation or diarrhea—may, in fact, be induced by the lack of synchronization between different body clocks.

It appears that we feel and do best when all of our internal clocks are synchronized with each other and with the cycles of day and night where we live. However, people differ as to how their sleep-wake cycles naturally cue with phases of light and dark outside. Evening people come alive at night, stay up into the wee hours of the morning, and sleep in long past sunrise whenever they can. Morning people, on the other hand, rise early, feel most alert in the morning, and go to bed soon after sunset, closing up like the leaves of the tamarind tree. Still others, probably the majority of us, lie somewhere between.[6] Each of us has an individual chronotype that describes the time of day our physical functions are most active.

Laypeople have often observed that plant species open their flowers at different times of day, just as bird species begin morning singing at different hours. In the United Kingdom, for example, the morning bird chorus may begin as early as 4:00 AM in the summer, starting with robins and blackbirds, followed by song thrushes, wrens, warblers, and house sparrows.[7] Where I live, in the high desert of New Mexico, flax and chicory bloom in the morning and usually close up by the time the poppies, peas, and daisies open, while my datura does not unwind its large tubular flowers until I am coming home from work, and their intoxicating aroma is strongest late at night. Variations like these exist within our own species, not only in the timing of our most alert hours but also in the length of our sleep, the ease of our waking, and even the difficulty of changing schedules.

These differences are not socially conditioned by work, school, or family schedules; they are biologically driven, though influenced by external circumstances, such as exposure to sunlight, work and school schedules, and family meal patterns. Ask any morning person what it is like trying to attend a concert that starts at 8:00 PM or a night person what it is like to get up before the sun. Hard as they may try, it is never easy, and they rarely get used to it. My mother, a night owl, used to go to meetings after dinner and leave my father, the morning bird in the family, home to watch us kids, though he inevitably fell asleep on the couch long before we did. Individual differences in the timing of sleep and waking exist regardless of ethnicity, gender, sociocultural position, and level of education. They are even found in flies and mice. It is increasingly clear that these different circadian settings, called chronotypes, are genetically influenced, biologically maintained, and hard to change, despite our best intentions.

Ever since assembly line production and cheap electrical light made it possible to run factories, employ shift workers, and keep university libraries open twenty-four hours a day, people have been trying to work and sleep at hours that are not of their choosing or nature. This mismatch between our internal biological rhythms and our actual sleep schedules (usually determined by school and work demands) has been given a name: social jet lag. Chronobiologist Till Roenneberg at Ludwig-Maximilians University in Munich, who coined the term, estimates that over 40 percent of the Central European population suffers from social jet lag of two hours or more.[8] Shift workers are particularly vulnerable. Currently, nearly 20 percent of employees in the industrialized world work evening, split, or rotating shifts.[9] Evening people are most suited to these schedules, and those with flexible circadian rhythms adjust pretty well, but many just cannot adapt and end up quitting.

They are probably the lucky ones. Research conducted since the 1990s has demonstrated that maintaining work and sleep schedules that conflict with one's internal circadian settings often exacts a hefty cost: persistent fatigue, digestive issues, and weight gain.[10] Many shift workers rely upon caffeine and sleeping pills, cigarettes and alcohol, to force wakefulness and sleep, further aggravating their social jet lag. A few years on rotating shifts puts them at greater risk of developing obesity, heart disease, depression, and ulcers.[11] To top it off, in 2007, the World Health

Organization listed "shift work that involves circadian disruption" as a possible carcinogen.[12] It is now clear that forcing oneself to fit into social schedules of school, work, and play against the grain of one's internal time will exact a price, sooner or later.

Being a lark, an owl, or a hummingbird that flits between the two is not a problem in itself, but ignoring internal rhythms to accommodate social clock time is a serious one. Since the turn of the twenty-first century, the American Academy of Sleep Medicine has identified a slew of new disorders: shift work disorder, advanced sleep phase disorder (when we fall asleep and wake up before the proper social time), delayed sleep phase disorder (when we fall asleep and wake up later than our jobs and schools request), jet lag disorder, excessive daytime sleepiness, and irregular sleep-wake rhythm.[13] As these manifestations of the tensions between individual biology and institutional regimes get labeled as medical disorders, the burden shifts from society at large onto the backs of individuals whose job it becomes to fix their so-called problems. Patients are given names for the difficulties they encounter with sleep, encouraged to get help, and the sleep industry swoops in to meet the ever-expanding need, offering everything from sleep concierges in high-end hotels to pharmaceutical wonder drugs.

While sleep medicine professionals have been adding new disorders to their list, researchers have been analyzing epidemiological data and publishing estimates of how much untreated sleep disorders cost society as a whole in terms of lost productivity, increased medical expenses, accidents, and mistakes.[14] The results have garnered a great deal of attention in the press, justifying the need for sleep medicine and catching the eye of a few large employers, such as Nike, Google, and Continental and British Airways, who now provide rest areas for their employees to improve performance. While it is sad to realize that the economic toll of sleep problems attracts more attention and response than the toll they take on our collective emotional and physical health, the issue has been gaining traction in the public arena.

Night Owls and Morning Larks

While it rarely works well to force a change of any kind in our circadian settings, our internal clocks do respond to the hormonal shifts that accompany critical points in the life cycle, such as puberty and menopause. It is now widely accepted that adolescence triggers a delay in the sleep-wake cycle, prompting teenagers to stay up—and wake up—later, much to the chagrin of parents and teachers.[15] The shift in sleep phase has been well documented throughout the industrialized world. In the 1990s, when pioneering researcher and psychiatrist Mary Carskadon followed a group of high school students as their school changed its start time from 8:25 AM to 7:20 AM, she noticed that nearly half became "pathologically sleepy" an hour into the school day, falling so quickly into REM sleep that they resembled narcoleptics.[16] The early start was so contrary to their biological rhythms it created sleep disorders where there were none before, an extreme case of social jet lag.

This night-owl phase shift explains why teens study and party so late, resist waking so strenuously, and shuffle like zombies between classes by day. They are not lazy, rebellious, or generally cantankerous. It is not television, video games, or texting that makes them that way. They simply sleep and wake to a different drummer, and the struggle to fit into school schedules is maddening to many. This biologically based time shift separates adolescents from adults, alienates them from society, and contributes to the creation of unique teen cultures. To some extent, every teen culture is a night culture, sharing the heretical thoughts and antiestablishment attitudes that have historically characterized those who prefer the evening hours, from medieval witches to eighteenth-century revolutionaries to twentieth-century jazz musicians.[17]

Inevitably, there comes a time when most young people settle down, as their parents put it, begin to wake up and go to bed earlier, give up their night-loving barista jobs, and take up daytime careers. In some societies, this shift in the timing of sleep-wake cycles is considered to mark the end of adolescence. However, some 10 percent of the population continues to prefer the evening throughout life, and they become lifelong night owls. A friend of mine once confided that the moment she retired from her eight-to-five job, she started staying up late, reading, writing, and drawing, just as she had done as an adolescent. She did not know it was still in her to be like that, and after years of forcing herself get up before dawn to cart the kids to school and drag herself to work on time, she was relieved to discover that she was not inherently dull or depressed. She was just a night person.

Unfortunately for night owls like my friend, most cultures favor, and often require, the early bird life. Aristotle instructed his followers that rising before dawn contributes to "health, wealth, and wisdom," words that were echoed centuries later by Benjamin Franklin in his famous proverb: "Early to bed, early to rise, makes a man healthy, wealthy, and wise." Religious teachers, be they Hindu, Buddhist, or Christian, encourage predawn rising for prayer and meditation. The Roman Catholic saint Josemaría Escrivá declared: "getting up on the dot, at a fixed time, without yielding a single minute to laziness" is "the heroic minute… If, with God's help, you conquer yourself, you will be ahead for the rest of the day." Then, in a moment of refreshing candor, he added: "It's so discouraging to find oneself beaten at the first skirmish!"[18]

It would be easy to conclude from these maxims that moral virtue is on the side of the early riser. Statistically, morning people outnumber night ones, so it may simply be a matter of majority rule. The preference could also stem from our agrarian roots before the invention of artificial light, when people needed to make full use of the daylight hours and protect themselves from predators at night. However, as the quotes above reveal, there is a righteousness attached to early rising, what author Robertson Davies called the "bony, blue-fingered hand of Puritanism"[19] that goes beyond these practicalities. In casting the effort we make to get up in the morning as a moral struggle against the tide of nature within us, cultures underscore the inherent difficulty of waking up, that strenuous labor that transforms us into socialized humans every morning.

A Body Tends to Stay at Rest

Scientists have a name for the struggle to wake up and get out of bed in the morning: sleep inertia.[20] Based on Newton's first law of motion (a body at rest tends to stay at rest), sleep inertia is most evident after an abrupt awakening from deep sleep, especially among those who are sleep deprived or naturally night loving. Some people, especially early risers, feel it the most after a short afternoon nap. It is that nearly irresistible desire to fall back asleep, when eyelids hang heavy and nothing else seems to matter, which explains why some people need four or five alarm clocks placed around the room to get themselves out of bed. I often have to give myself a stern talk to muster up motivation for the day because I do not care about anything—or anyone—those first few minutes. Sleep inertia is a mixture of sleeping and waking states characterized by grogginess, clumsiness, and fleeting disorientation.

It appears that our brains do not switch on like lightbulbs the moment we wake, even though it may seem so at times. Parts of our brains activate more quickly and fully than others, and tasks that require timely coordination between the parts, such as walking downstairs or answering questions, often falter.[21]

While sleep inertia has undoubtedly been a part of the human experience throughout the ages, its symptoms were first noted scientifically in the 1950s, when it was found that Air Force pilots stationed in their cockpits for quick takeoff were more apt to make mistakes during the first five to twenty minutes after being woken from sleep.[22] Research has since demonstrated that memory, manual dexterity, and complex decision making suffer under the spell of sleep inertia.[23] The effects are, as one researcher put it, "as bad or worse than being legally drunk" and roughly equivalent to going without sleep for seventy hours.[24] It takes longer to perform the simplest of tasks, like finding the milk in the refrigerator. Accidents are more common. Even our capacity to do simple math declines.

We might ask: who makes important calculations the moment they wake up? Emergency responders, soldiers, firefighters, and medical personnel are routinely woken from sleep and required to respond immediately to critical situations. They make decisions and perform procedures that can save—or lose—lives, including their own, within the first few minutes. Since they are not usually fully awake, emergency responders come to rely on habits developed and perfected over years of practice, which usually serve them quite well. But when faced with complex decisions, and already sleep deprived from working long hours and changing shifts, those habits may not suffice. Fortunately, most of us get to stretch, yawn, and drink a cup of coffee or tea before we turn our focus to the world around us—or take lives into our hands. I have always assumed that I am safely in command of my abilities by the time I get behind the wheel to go to work, but it turns out I have been wrong. Research indicates that many of us do not reach our full abilities for two hours after waking, something I try to remember in morning traffic.[25]

Sleep inertia would not be a problem if we did not make such demands upon our every waking minute of our days—if we did not drive cars, perform emergency surgeries, run into burning houses, or take off on bombing missions within minutes of waking. One has to wonder why we do these things. Why schedule firefighters and medical interns for thirty-hour shifts, forcing them to catnap when things are quiet, only to be suddenly woken by a fire alarm or a code blue? Why put their lives—and ours—at such unnecessary risk? I suspect it has something to do with our human desire to push the limits of our abilities, to excel and exceed, to be superhuman. It also displays our cultural preference for wakefulness. *Preference* may be too mild a term, for waking awareness is considered by many to be the only form of consciousness of any value. It has become the gold standard by which all other states of mind are measured, which explains why scientists are funded to wake subjects from sound sleep and test their abilities to keep their eyes open, do math, remember things, and think quickly—all measures of waking alertness—only to decry how poorly they perform. Why not test for mental flexibility, emotional receptivity or creativity, qualities that emerge at the soft edges and lapses of waking focus?

It is like evaluating the quality of light at dawn or dusk by the standard of the blazing midday sun and finding it lacking. The subtlety, richness, and depth of transitional states are ignored altogether in favor of the speed, focus, and hypervigilance of heightened alertness the world seems to demand of us. Drowsiness, that mixed state of waking and sleeping modes of awareness, is at best dismissed and at worst demeaned as a medical disorder in need of treatment, a liability at work and school, even a moral failure.

Where the Two Worlds Touch

There are people who treasure morning drowsiness, allowing themselves to drift in and out of sleep for the sheer pleasure of it. I have heard it described as sleep-surfing and zauzzling in the vernacular of urban slang, described as something we do on days off when we don't have to get out of bed right away and get to lay there "half asleep and half awake at the same time." You might hear an intruder downstairs when there is none, wonder why it is light outside when you are sure it is nighttime, or talk out loud to a dream character. Sometimes voices are heard or presences felt. Charles Dickens described it well:

> There is a kind of sleep which steals upon us sometimes… and yet we have consciousness of all that is going on about us, and even if we dream, words which are really spoken, or sounds which really exist at the moment, accommodate themselves with surprising readiness to our visions, until reality and imagination become so strangely blended.[26]

Scientists consider this to be Stage 1 sleep, but if you ask someone if she is sleeping, she will probably deny it.

Dickens was describing what could be called a quasi-lucid dream because he was consciously awake and dreaming simultaneously, an experience many have had from time to time. Lucid dreaming is a natural talent for some, and a cultivated skill for others, that has been developed in cultures around the world, from the Himalayan Mountains to the highlands of Central America to the Arctic Circle.[27] Starting with an intention to wake up, or stay awake, while dreaming, lucid dreamers eventually develop the ability to explore worlds, gather new knowledge, and facilitate healing for themselves and others. In some Hindu and Buddhist traditions, practitioners learn to observe their dreams from a distance and consciously interact with them as a meditation tool that can be applied to waking life as well.[28] I have heard this practice referred to as night school. Transitional states between sleep and waking provide fertile ground for the night school of lucid dreaming, whether intentional or accidental.

Stage 1 sleep is characterized by large alpha and theta brain waves, frequencies associated with a relaxed, more inwardly focused awareness. Theta waves, in particular, can access information beyond our ordinary awareness, such as distant memories, intuitive insights, or answers to puzzles we have been pondering. Mystics describe it as a time when the door between worlds swings open, which is why Rumi advised in his poem "Unseen Rain":

> The breeze at dawn has secrets to tell you.
> Don't go back to sleep.
> You must ask for what you really want.
> Don't go back to sleep.
> People are going back and forth across the doorsill
> Where the two worlds touch.
> The door is round and open.
> Don't go back to sleep.[29]

In work-oriented cultures, people often have to rush through the transitions between waking and sleeping to keep up with the demands of life. Desperate for more shut-eye, we try to fall asleep and wake up as quickly as possible to get the most out of our time in bed. If it takes twenty or thirty minutes to drop off—which sleep experts tell us is normal—many wonder what is wrong and resort to alcohol or pills to speed things along. In fact, sleep scientists consider the rapidity with which we slip in and out of sleep to be a measure of what they call sleep efficiency.[30] An efficient sleeper spends over 90 percent of his or her time in bed asleep, spending as little time awake as possible.

We are supposed to take the fast elevators, the ones that drop like stones and rise like rockets, between sleeping and waking, not the slow ones that carry us through the shades between, where communion occurs and each state absorbs some of the other. "We have all learned to carry out this exercise in self-impoverishment… " observed psychologist Ann Faraday years ago. "The alarm rings, and instantaneously an axe falls across the continuum of consciousness, sharply dividing wake from sleep."[31]

When morning coffees and evening nightcaps hasten the passage, they further divide and polarize the worlds we inhabit by day and by night, making it harder to carry experience from one into the other. Things drop into the waters of forgetting, the River Lethe that surrounds the cave of sleep in ancient Greek mythology. As a result, our waking and dreaming lives proceed unbeknownst to each other, like continents slowly drifting apart.

The biochemical changes that accompany our passages do not make it easy to remember one world while entering the next. We forget almost every time, crashing into the next world as if the last one never existed. Is it a biological imperative, unwitting negligence, or the better part of wisdom to plunge ourselves into the waters of oblivion when traveling between sleeping and waking worlds?

The ancient Greeks considered it to be a case of carelessness, for they called Lethe *ameles potamos*, the "river of unmindfulness." In their view, it is not inevitable that we forget one world upon entering the next, but a simple lack of attention. Hindu philosophers remind us that we do not have to be unconscious in sleep; we simply allow it to be that way out of spiritual laziness, for lack of a better term.[32] If we allowed ourselves to pause and drift, to zauzzle, in the passage between states, we would find it much easier to carry experiences across the divide.

Many traditional cultures hold nightlong healing ceremonies that, in effect, use sleep deprivation to cultivate drowsiness and weave the worlds of sleep and waking back together, if only temporarily. Participants nod in and out as they fight to stay awake, and I suspect their trance-like sleepiness is instrumental to the work of the ritual, be it the Navajo Night Chant, the Balinese Hindu Shivaratri, or the Peruvian Ayahuasca ceremony. Hindus identify a fourth state of consciousness beneath and beyond waking, dreaming, and deep sleep, an impersonal witnessing awareness that exists at the juncture of all three.[33] All-night ritual observances may take us close to that fourth state: beyond tired but still awake, consciously engaged in a shared dream, while watching it all from afar. At times like this, we lose our sense of certainty, self-possession, and resistance to the unfamiliar within and without us. Things become capable of changing.

The world itself seems strangely liquid and transitory, and we are quick to realize that things may not be what we think they are. Questions arise where there were none before. It can be disorienting, even frightening, without a ritual structure to contain the confusion. One could say that sleepiness is a ground for transformation, one to be cherished, guarded, and approached with respect. In the right hands, it is an avenue of healing. However, when we stay up longer to get more done, stealing hours from our sleep and forcing rapid transitions, we may forgo that opportunity for healing.

16

ENAMORED WITH WAKEFULNESS: PHASING OUT SLEEP

It has been said that there are two kinds of people: those that damn the world for interfering with their sleep and those who damn their bodies for needing sleep. Similarly, there are two ways to respond to the biological need for sleep: one can take pills to get more of it or take pills to require less of it. As Jefferson Airplane famously sang: "One pill makes you larger, and one pill makes you small."[1]

A few years back, when I was visiting with a smart, young psychiatrist at the end of his workday at a local community health center, I mentioned that I still struggled with tiredness, even though I had mostly recovered from chronic fatigue syndrome (CFS). He listened attentively, tapping away on his computer to make notes of our conversation, and occasionally spinning around to look up something in one of the medical textbooks on the shelf behind him. He told me there was a new drug on the market called Provigil that was showing promising results for people with CFS, relieving the worst of its mind-numbing exhaustion. I did not pursue the topic at the time because I was not looking to take more medication, but I remember marveling at his energy, quick mind, and avid interest, especially because he told me afterward that his wife had had twins the week before, and they were keeping them up all night, every night.

At the time, I wrote off his electric vitality to youth, first-time fatherhood, and the rigorous training of medical school, all of which left me feeling old, weary, sloppy, and slow. But since I have begun to hear and read about what are being called the new smart drugs, including Provigil (the brand name for modafinil), it has occurred to me that this young doctor was probably a living demonstration of their effectiveness.

Cities of Gold

Provigil was originally developed in France by neurophysiologist and early sleep researcher Michel Jouvet for the treatment of narcolepsy, and it was launched with FDA approval as a prescription medication in the United States in 1999.[2] It is a mood-brightening, memory-enhancing, wakefulness-promoting drug that can keep people alert for two days without the jitters of caffeine, the mood swings of amphetamines, or sleep debt accumulation. It simply puts off the need for sleep for a couple of days, with few side effects.

The promise of Provigil is so attractive, so sexy, that observers have dubbed Provigil "Viagra for the brain," and it can be easily purchased online without prescription. Everyone who wants or needs to stay awake for a long time has found his or her dreams come true in this little, pricey pill. Even though scientists are unsure at this time how Provigil works, undecided as to whether it is addictive, and clueless about the long-term effects, sales are well over $1 billion a year.[3] Provigil's vast underground popularity reveals the extent to which we value wakefulness, dislike drowsiness, and avoid sleep.

These predilections did not arise overnight. Stimulants have played a vital role in human societies since the beginning. There have always been times when people needed to stay awake and alert to protect loved ones, travel long distances, hunt, harvest crops, or fight battles. The Mayans had chocolate; the Chinese, tea; South Americans, guarana; West Africans, kola nuts; and South Asians, betal leaves.[4] But Europeans were not exposed to caffeine until the fifteenth and sixteenth centuries, when explorers, crusaders, and traders brought back the three great drug foods—coffee, tea, and chocolate—from distant lands. A century later, there were more than three thousand coffeehouses in England alone, where men (women were not allowed) exchanged news, debated politics, and brokered deals into the wee hours of the morning. One of the earliest coffeehouses in England advertised that coffee would "prevent drowsiness and make one fit for business."

In the heated frenzy of the European coffeehouses of the sixteenth and seventeenth centuries, merchants devised our modern systems of credit and speculation to fund oversees explorations in search of legendary cities of gold. Lloyd's of London insurance market originated in a London coffeehouse by that name. As caffeine rushed through the merchants' veins, increasing heart rates, dilating pupils, tightening muscles, and boosting confidence, traders arranged to put off paying for their risky enterprises while the coffee they ingested postponed their need to sleep. Their dealings laid the foundation for European colonialism and international slave trade, which used people of color and foreign lands to produce stimulants—tea, coffee, sugar, and tobacco—for a ravenous white European market.

Stimulants ushered in the Age of Enlightenment, when sleep was increasingly characterized as a form of slothful indulgence, and waking busyness a form of moral rectitude. Proverbs instructed people with veiled threats: "In the morning, be the first up, and in the evening last to go to bed, for they that sleep catch no fish." "He who sleeps all morning through will end up begging in the afternoon." My favorite, though, comes from Thomas Edison, who brought electric lights into American streets and homes, extending productive hours by pushing back the limits of darkness. He wrote in his diary: "Most people overeat 100 percent, and oversleep 100 percent, because they like it. That extra 100 percent makes them unhealthy and inefficient. The person who sleeps eight to ten hours a night is never fully asleep and never fully awake—they have only different degrees of dozing through the twenty-four hours."

Sleepy, Dopey, Bashful, and Grumpy

Edison epitomized what could be called the culture of productivity that valorizes the qualities of wakefulness: activity, alertness, speed, and efficiency. His disdain for dozing reveals an assumption held by many in the northern latitudes: that the hours of our days are intended for labor, not for sleepy daydreaming or rocking babies. Northern Europeans and Americans consume four times the amount of caffeine on a daily basis than Africans or Asians do.[5] Ever since Walt Disney named the seven dwarfs in *Snow White* in 1937, Sleepy has been kin to Dopey, Sneezy, Bashful, and Grumpy in the Western world. Even though drowsiness is a natural transitional phase in the human cycles of rest and activity, it has come to be seen as dimwitted, sluggish, negligent, and even dangerous. Coffee is so much a part of work life that the breaks we are guaranteed by law every four hours are commonly called coffee breaks, and most every office has a pot brewing all day, not to mention vending machines with caffeinated energy drinks like Mountain Dew and Red Bull. Stimulants have become the "boss's little helpers," as journalist David Plotz so aptly put it.[6] They help us work harder and better.

Many stimulants are now called smart drugs, neuro-enhancers, and cognitive-enhancing drugs, a class that includes everything from a cup of coffee to Provigil, with amphetamines like Benzedrine, Ritalin, and Adderall in between. No longer restricted to the treatment of asthma, narcolepsy, and attention-deficit disorder, smart drugs are commonly used by students, soldiers, academics, medical personnel, entrepreneurs, investment bankers, musicians, executives, and even professional poker players to improve their drive, focus, thinking, and stamina. One executive explained that he took Adderall to "continue the lightning pace and constant multitasking his job requires."[7] Two neuroscientists, Barbara Sahakian and Sharon Morein-Zamir, admitted in an interview for *Nature* magazine, "We know that a number of our scientific colleagues in the United States and the United Kingdom already use modafinil to counteract the effects of jetlag, to enhance productivity or mental energy, or to deal with demanding and important intellectual challenges."[8] *Nature* magazine titled their commentary on modafinil "professor's little helper."

As we raise the bar of what we expect of ourselves during our waking hours, anything less becomes a problem to be treated, a failing that must be addressed. The popular saying, "You snooze, you lose," expresses the increasingly prevalent notion that if you miss something in a lapse of attention, you will go down without a second chance like the Olympian runner who stumbles out of the block. Accordingly, sleep medicine now defines subwakefulness syndrome (otherwise known as excessive daytime sleepiness) as a clinical disorder, and in 2004 in the US the FDA approved modafinil for a variety of syndromes associated with excessive daytime sleepiness.[9] While there are some professions that truly demand long hours of sharp focus, such as surgery, most of us do not risk anyone's life when our attention drifts. We can allow ourselves to cycle between phases of rest and activity, diffuse and pointed awareness, as our biology requires.

However, students and professionals are beginning to feel pressure to use neuro-enhancing drugs when their peers are taking them, just to keep up. The use of so-called smart drugs (it is not clear whether they actually make us any smarter) has spread like wildfire because it promises a competitive edge but also because people fear they will be left in the dust if they do not take them. Whether or not that fear is founded, its prevalence exposes the tremendous pressure that many feel to perform at top-notch levels day in and day out. Studies have shown that anywhere from 5 to 35 percent of college students use stimulants, and they usually continue taking them as young professionals.[10] When *Wired* magazine surveyed its readers after reporting on professor's little helper, many responded by detailing the brain-enhancing regimes they have developed, often combining amphetamines with modafinil.[11]

The United States military, understandably, leads the way in sleep-replacement research. After all, soldiers sometimes have to go for three or four days with little or no sleep, and their lives depend on their ability to stay alert, focused, and cool headed. In 2002, the Pentagon's Defense Advanced Research Projects Agency (DARPA) called for a "radical approach" to attain "continuous assisted performance" for up to a week, beyond what stimulants like caffeine and amphetamines can offer.[12] Retired Rear Admiral Stephen Baker, with the Center for Defense Information, called it the "better warrior through chemistry" approach.

While militaries have dispensed amphetamines to soldiers in almost every war since World War II, the side effects of hypertension, mood swings, and addiction have posed serious problems. In 2003, US Air Force Majors William Umbach and Harry Schmidt were court-martialed after mistakenly dropping a bomb that killed four Canadian soldiers in Afghanistan.[13] During the pretrial hearing, one of their attorneys disclosed that the pilots were pressured by superiors to take "go pills" (amphetamines) before flying, and the defendants believed the medication impaired their judgment. Even though charges were dropped, the revelation that Air Force pilots flying F-16 bombers routinely took amphetamines sparked public outrage. Incidents like this further motivated DARPA to test modafinil. The drug had already been employed by the French during the first Gulf War, and the United States Air Force had tested it on pilots flying forty-hour sorties during Operation Enduring Freedom in Afghanistan.

At this point, our culture of productivity is racing toward a forty-eight-hour day—or at least seriously entertaining the fantasy. Researchers and observers alike predict that sleep will become controllable and dispensable in ten to twenty years through cosmetic neurology, the steady supply of stimulating and sedating drugs that will enable us to sleep and wake at will. Russell Foster, a circadian biologist at Imperial College London, predicted that "in ten to twenty years we'll be able to pharmacologically turn sleep off. Mimicking sleep will take longer, but I can see it happening."[14] To those who question this direction, or its momentum, researchers respond that we are already living in a society that is self-medicating with coffee, alcohol, energy drinks, and sleeping pills to shift gears on an hourly basis.[15] We are already hooked into the stimulant-sedation loop. Why not develop and use better means, with fewer side effects, to control our biological need for rest?

It is a good question, and one for which I have no clear answer, only a few thoughts about what's at stake. We know sleep benefits our physical and emotional health; presumably it would continue to do so whether we get to it tonight or three nights from now. What I worry about is the trouble we could get ourselves into in the meantime, while we speed ahead full throttle without intervals of sleepiness to reflect, imagine possible consequences, and question what we are doing or intermissions of sleep to help us regroup and come up with better solutions. Deep sleep and dreaming help "set the stage for the emergence of insight," as neuroscientist Ullrich Wagner and his colleagues demonstrated and explained.[16] Without regular, recurring opportunities for insight, we could become blinded by our own drives—like my dog, who cannot hear approaching cars—or our frantic calls—when she is chasing after something.

There is a particular blind spot that comes with the regular use of stimulants that has been evident throughout history, from the coffeehouses of seventeenth-century Europe to those of twentieth-century Silicon Valley. It is related to their dopamine-centered mood-brightening effect (my favorite of all their gifts) and shows itself as an effervescent brilliance and an unshakable faith in one's vision. One internet proponent of modafinil calls himself the "bulletproof executive;" another titled his piece, "How I Became Mighty with Modafinil." This exhilarating sense of mission carries along with it a propensity to ignore problems, pull fast ones, and whitewash ethical lapses as long as one can get away with them. It reminds me of careening down the ski slopes, barely in control and hanging on for dear life. The shaky doubts and ethical questions of sobriety are no match for the speed and power of the ride.

Cephalon, the small pharmaceutical company that purchased and marketed Provigil in the United States, exemplified these risks and rewards, in my opinion. Founded in 1987 to pursue treatments for neurodegenerative diseases, Cephalon grew to become one of the top ten biotechnology firms in the world with $2.8 billion in annual revenues in twenty-five short years.[17] It was an astounding accomplishment, and it did so, in part, by continually creating new markets for Provigil, getting the FDA to approve additional uses, and advertising even more widespread ones, such as daytime sleepiness. However, the company was also sued for off-label marketing, price-fixing, and antitrust violations, prompting *Businessweek* magazine to announce: "This Pep Pill Is Pushing Its Luck."[18] But the most egregious crime, in the eyes of many, was conspiring with potential generic manufacturers of Provigil to keep generics off the market and make consumers continue to pay high prices, what FTC Chairman Jon Leibowitz called "one of the worst abuses across the board in health care."[19]

Cephalon's growth was unfettered and unscrupulous, a bubble waiting to burst. It has become my image for what can happen when we banish the input of regular sleep. As Sir Thomas Browne once observed, "We term sleep a death; and yet it is waking that kills us." However, one example does not make a case, and this case may not be worth making. It reminds me of the dire predictions that are often made when a new technology is introduced into our daily lives. People worried that radios would disturb the silence and artificial lights would banish darkness. Well, they have, and we adapted, so who cares?

I would rather argue that the popularity of both stimulants and sedatives suggests that we have lost our tolerance for sleepiness—that half-awake/half-asleep state that ushers us between the extremes of sleep and waking. We take pills to shorten the time it takes to fall asleep and then drink coffee to speed our delivery into the waking world. Why must we dash through those in-between places where the realms we inhabit by day and by night collide, converse, and occasionally collaborate?

I catch myself eating chocolate after lunch to pick myself up for the afternoon and listening to my iPod when I wake at night to speed my way back into sleep, as if I needed to keep my day and night worlds pure and separate, despite my knowledge of the fruitful "quiet wakefulness" that psychiatrist Thomas A. Wehr's subjects experienced when waking between sleeps. When I look honestly, I would have to say that broken sleep and waking drowsiness, those disturbing mixtures of waking and sleeping, seem somehow wrong and even bad to me, though I do not know why. I move instinctually to prevent, erase and cover those bouts the way we hold our hands over our mouths when we yawn, or look away when we come upon someone sleeping on the sidewalk. It is one of those unspoken, underlying cultural beliefs I learned without ever knowing it: there is something uncouth and dangerous that occurs at the intersection of sleep and waking.

There's a lot of money being made off that discomfort. Personally, I would rather learn to take my time falling asleep, wake slowly, dawdle dimwitted for a while the next morning, enjoy short shut-eyes in the afternoon whenever I can, and save the pills for when I really need them.

17

WAKING UP AGAIN: DOUBT, CERTAINTY, AND THE FUTURE OF SLEEP

Have you ever woken up, looked at the clock, and prepared for the day, only to wake up again and realize that the first time was a dream? It is a fairly common occurrence, sometimes called a false awakening or a double dream. Philosopher Bertrand Russell reported having about a hundred of these in a row while coming round from a general anesthetic. It reminds me of those Russian nesting dolls that open up to reveal another doll nestled inside, which opens up to reveal yet another one, and so forth. What interests me about these experiences is how similar the dreamed waking life is to the physical one. They both present believable worlds, primarily visual ones, with a sense of self in the center taking action. The similarity begs the question: what isn't merely perception?

The Subliminal Storehouse of Consciousness

We know that what we see, hear, feel, smell, and taste is only a fraction of what exists out there. Dogs can hear and smell things we cannot. Birds and insects see things we cannot. Some animals detect electrical and magnetic fields. Dolphins use sonar to find their way. What we experience of the world around us is actually a portrait created by our brains from the limited information given by our senses at any moment in time of an infinitely richer physical reality. Our brains constantly scan for recognizable patterns by which to identify what is out there, relying upon memory and knowledge (what scientists call our schemas) to categorize and conceptualize. We could even say that we inhabit virtual realities formed from the splatters of sensory input we receive, in which the blanks are filled in by what we know from past experience. It is a continual creation that is so seamless, we do not even realize we are looking at pictures rather than the world itself.

I own a small painting that reminds me of this continual creation. It has curving streaks of purples, greens, pinks, oranges, black, and white that—when viewed as a whole from more than a few feet away—look like the surface of a pond after someone has thrown a stone in. No piece or part of the painting looks anything like water, but my brain reads this arrangement of colors and lines as just that, even with a story attached of what happened a moment before. It seems that, having observed rippling water many times, my mind holds an image or schema of what it looks like and, finding similarities with this pattern of curving colors, automatically imposes its picture so I can recognize what the painting is about. The overlay happens so quickly, I do not even notice it. Our unconscious minds automatically interpret sensory input from our stores of previous experiences, all the while fooling us into believing we are actually seeing what is there.

While I am not a religious scholar, I suspect it is these stored patterns of experience that compose what Buddhist and Hindu texts refer to as the illusions of both dreaming and waking life. In the Advaita school of Hinduism, ignorance is composed of two actions: not seeing something for what it is (*tattva jnana*) and perceiving it as something else (*anayatha-grahana*).[1] It is a dual process of nonapprehension and misapprehension that prompts us to mistake that rope for a snake or a shell for a piece of silver, and this occurs all the time, whether we are awake or asleep and dreaming. The Mahayana Buddhist tradition posits the existence of a subliminal storehouse of consciousness (*alaya vijnana*) that contains traces, or impressions, of all past experience.[2] Teachers in this tradition explain that we constantly project these traces onto the world around us without thinking, convincing ourselves that they have a concrete, independent existence when they do not. They are illusions, appearances we are constantly creating in that dual process of nonapprehension and misapprehension. The Hindu word for these illusions is *maya*. Buddhists call them reifications, abstractions that are mistakenly considered to have material reality.

It is a heady notion. The concept baffled me for some time, until a friend gave me an example: race. Biologically, there is no such thing as race; no clear basis to categorize human beings into different groups. The idea was developed in the context of imperialist ventures over many centuries, socially and legally enforced and reinforced so often that we have come to collectively believe it has a concrete reality. Race has become a central feature of identity, social structure, and political discourse, generating enormous suffering on all sides. But it is just an abstract notion, no more real or tangible than any other idea.

Some of these unconscious traces, what contemporary cognitive psychologists would call schemas, are emotionally charged and fueled by painful past experiences, while others are more detached assumptions we learn almost by osmosis. Either way, these are the beliefs and identities we hold near and dear, the smudges that obscure the Clear Light Mind, to use the Buddhist term. They give rise to the world that appears to us, entangling us in dramas day and night, which is why these traditions see little difference between dreaming and waking experience. As Carl Jung observed, even in waking life, we "continue to dream beneath the threshold of consciousness."[3]

Neuroscientists are beginning to agree. Rodolfo Llinás, who studies what happens in the brain during different states of consciousness, has proposed that our dreaming and waking minds are not distinct but are aspects of the same intrinsic brain functions. "Wakefulness," he wrote, "is nothing other than a dreamlike state modulated by... sensory inputs."[4] In other words, our senses place us in time and space; without their input, we would be continuously dreaming. Dr. V. S. Ramachandran offered another explanation based on his study of visual illusions: "In a sense, we are all hallucinating all the time. What we call normal vision is our selecting the hallucination that best fits reality."[5]

As we go about our days and nights selecting among hallucinations, something guides our choices. When we are awake and receiving information from our senses about the temperature outside, the amount of light around us, our bodies' positions in space, and so on, the options are limited to a few possibilities. We make our best guesses and reify them, treating them as if they had concrete existence. When we are asleep and dreaming, cut off from awareness of our surroundings, something else directs those choices. Latent traces, subtle impressions, or internalized schemas may steer the stories that unfold in our dreams, or they may simply frame the perception and interpretation of random neuronal firings. Either way, our experiences are immediately reified, for the lives we lead behind closed eyelids seem as real and believable as our waking ones. Once we open our eyes, these same traces most likely continue to provide the basis for what we perceive, but within the range of what our senses tell us.

In the end, we are left with the quandary Henry David Thoreau articulated so well nearly two hundred years ago: "I do not know how to distinguish between our waking life and a dream. Are we not always living the life that we imagine we are?" Of course we are. The realization itself triggers another sort of awakening by prompting us to question our ordinary, habitual perceptions. But in practical terms, when we hop in the car and start driving, we need to know we are awake and responding to cars and traffic lights that truly exist. How can we tell? The French novelist Marcel Proust offered a clue when he wrote of waking one morning: "I was now well awake; my body had veered round for the last time and the good angel of certainty had made all the surrounding objects stand still, and had set me down… in my bedroom."

The Good Angel of Certainty

Clarity, stability, and familiarity. These are the qualities we come to rely upon in our waking lives—the criteria we most often use to decide that we are, in fact, awake and not dreaming. With Proust's "good angel of certainty," we reconstitute ourselves and our lives every time we wake up. When I first open my eyes, I look around to see where I am, then glance outside or at the clock to learn the time, figure out what day it is, and go about retrieving from memory what I have to do that day. If I wake up in an unfamiliar place or at a strange time, it takes me longer to get my bearings and piece myself together. If I am hungover, sick, or stirred by a strong dream, the confusion can last longer. There is a fleeting cacophony of sensations as my nightlife mingles with my day world. But eventually certainty arrives, convincing me that the world I see is real, and I am able to get up and begin my day.

Certainty, that habit of believing we know (even if we do not) is essential for our survival in the waking world. We need to trust that the flash of red we see to the right of the street is a stoplight in order to brake in time to avoid being hit; we do not have the luxury to ask ourselves whether we are dreaming or imagining it. But that same certainty, an unmitigated confidence in our perceptions, is also one of the greatest liabilities of waking consciousness. It convinces us we are right, hardens our beliefs, and solidifies our prejudices, inevitably giving rise to conflict with others. As the English critic Terry Eagleton observed: "If it is true that we need a degree of certainty to get by, it is also true that too much of the stuff can be lethal."[6]

Without a corrective dose of doubt to prompt us to question assumptions, listen to other points of view, and consider alternate courses of action, we are in trouble, as individuals and as nations. Former president Bill Clinton appeared to agree when he mentioned in a question-and-answer session following a speech he gave at the University of California in Berkeley in 2007: "One of the reasons that there is often such an acrimonious atmosphere in Washington, is that too many members of the Congress in both parties are sleep deprived… And it clouds your judgment, and it undermines your ability to be relaxed and respectful in dealing with your adversaries."[7] Alluding to both the cognitive and emotional tolls that sleeplessness incurs, Clinton implies that conflicts could be better handled, and even resolved, if everyone involved got enough sleep. The cause of peace would do well to put sleep on its agenda.

Sleep is, as Shakespeare's Macbeth noted, the "balm of hurt minds." We need those hours of slumber to interrupt our string of days, unravel our convictions, soften our hearts, and return us to life's underside of fluid confusion. With this understanding, the transition from sleeping to waking becomes important because it allows the life we lead behind closed eyes to inform our waking activity. It fosters the patience, respect, and flexibility, what some would call wisdom, required to address our most pressing problems.

The Future of Sleep

When I first moved to New Mexico some thirty years ago, I befriended an older neighbor whose family had lived in the area for generations. Antonio had worked in the molybdenum mine up the road for many years until he was injured and forced to retire, which gave him plenty of time to watch CNN, observe the ways of the world, and educate newcomers like me. He told me about the Moorish origins of the local acequia system that Spaniards integrated with existing American Indian irrigation systems in the 1600s to equitably collect, conserve, and distribute runoff from the mountains. Water is a precious resource in the high arid desert, and Antonio never took it for granted. He washed his truck by hand on the small patch of grass he grew for his baby grandson so the runoff would keep it green. He remembered what it was like before the fences went up, when you could walk everywhere and drink any running water.

All that changed when the railroad came to Albuquerque, Antonio explained, bringing Anglo-Americans who soon imposed their ways, their language, and their laws. Land that had been communally owned under Spanish law was appropriated, legally and illegally, under American law, often without the knowledge or consent of the previous owners. "Before long," Antonio added, "they were selling our land back to us."

When a ski resort was developed upstream, with a sewage plant near the headwaters of the creek that ran through our valley, the water became unsafe to drink. The hand-dug wells that Antonio and his neighbors relied upon for household water dried up. When Antonio complained, the city fathers told him he would have to hook up to city water or dig a deeper well. Antonio was fed up: "Now they're selling our water back to us. Before you know it," he added, shaking his finger at me, "they'll be selling the air back to us."

When buying bottled water became the everyday norm, I thought of Antonio, relieved that he was no longer alive to see his predictions come true. Despite everything he taught me, I was amazed to discover how easily we relinquished our right to clean water, how willing we have been to pay for something that had been free and available from every fountain, faucet, and creek a few short years ago. When oxygen bars popped up in the cities, I wanted to run over to Antonio's house, show him the newspaper article, and say, "Antonio, you were right; they're selling our air back to us." I wanted to hear that long whistle of his.

Now, they are selling our sleep back to us. Sleep used to be so easy that most people ignored it and took it for granted. Now, good sleep is hard to come by, and people worry about getting it, losing it, not getting enough of it, and having to do without it. Like clean water, fresh air, and the other endangered resources of our natural world, we are just beginning to appreciate the sleep that is vanishing before our eyes.

As of the writing of this book, a new class of sleep medication is seeking approval in the US.[8] Developed by neuroscientists working at the Merck Research Laboratories in West Point, DORA-22 (also known by its brand name, Suvorexant) has been shown to facilitate sleep in monkeys without causing the grogginess and cognitive impairment commonly associated with previous sleeping pills. It works by targeting a different receptor in the brain, shutting down wakefulness rather than cultivating sleepiness.

While early trials on humans were promising, increasing the total amount of sleep, an FDA advisory panel raised concerns about side effects of daytime drowsiness and suicidal thinking, and requested lower dosages in May of 2013. The FDA appears to be exercising more caution this time around, and questions certainly remain about the safety of the new drug. As physician and sleep researcher Christian Guilleminault, who played a central role in the discovery and treatment of obstructive sleep apnea, noted in reference to DORA-22, "When you have something new you don't know everything you would like to know."[9] Even so, the public relations people at Merck are spreading the word and building excitement for their new drug, and almost every major news outlet has already featured it. We are heading down that well-worn primrose path again, the road every other sleeping pill has taken, from barbiturates to benzodiazepines to the nonbenzodiazepines that just arrived, in our insatiable desire for quick and easy sleep.

Meanwhile, military-funded scientists have found a drug that "eliminates sleepiness," and it works with the same brain receptors as DORA-22, only in reverse.[10] A simple nasal spray, Orexin-A, is being touted as a promising candidate for sleep replacement because it reduces drowsiness and maintains waking levels of cognition in monkeys without the edginess, increased blood pressure, and mood swings associated with amphetamines. It is readily available on the internet, even though the spray has not been formally tested on humans yet, remains years away from FDA approval as of 2013, and may not relieve or prevent any of the other effects of sleep deprivation. One of the researchers involved in the study, Jerome Siegel, warned: "You'd have to be a fool to advocate taking this and reducing sleep as much as possible."[11]

Siegel knows what people want. The fantasy of reducing and manipulating sleep to suit our desires is alive and well, and the reality may not be far off, though I suspect that problems will arise—as they tend to do in the pursuit of this fantasy—reminding us that we are still creatures like all the rest who inhabit this earth. In the end, the problem is not with the pharmaceutical companies or the sleep industry, both of which meet a need as much they create one, but with the cultural values that lie beneath the entire phenomenon: the drive to control nature as it exists within and without us. For sleep is, if nothing else, one of nature's ways, and it remains as indispensable to life as eating. Much as we might want to domesticate our slumber, sleep is both wild and indigenous to this planet.

I suspect that sleep has its own reasons to be, ones that elude the scientists who continue to scratch their heads and wonder why we do it. Researchers have contributed immensely to our knowledge of the ways sleep sustains the waking side of our lives, renewing our physical, mental, and emotional health, and they will probably find more. They have done such a good job that sleep is beginning to be viewed as a performance enhancer, especially by athletes and progressive employers. Hopefully this knowledge will help return sleep to its rightful place in our lives and world, and begin to reverse our acceptance of shortened, disrupted sleep as the way of life. However, it also projects a future in which sleep itself is commoditized for commercial aims in the name of progress.

But what does the future of sleep look like from sleep's perspective? Over the course of researching and writing this book, I have come to think of sleep in our day and age as a wild creature that has been taken into captivity, trying desperately to adapt to a radically changed habitat. It is alive but struggling, showing signs of stress from the effort to adjust to new and constraining conditions: impossible schedules, nighttime lights, overseas flights, a chemical soup of stimulants and sedatives, and hypervigilant nervous systems, to name a few. Tigers in captivity pace in their cages, elephants rock back and forth, and many of us act like narcoleptics, falling asleep at work and in the car but lying awake fretting for hours in the night. We have come to accept these behaviors as ordinary, even normal, but they are neither appropriate nor healthy. They are signs of distress.

We do not have to live this way. We may not be able to turn the tide of history, but we can change the conditions under which we sleep. Just as zookeepers have learned to provide ample room, familiar habitats, and preferred company to suit the animals they house, we can adapt our environments, work, and family cultures to foster restorative sleep. It is simply a matter of shifting our focus from the demands of our days to the needs—and offerings—of our nights under the covers.

It has become increasingly clear that our sleep shapes who we are as much, if not more, than we shape it. Sleep colors our perceptions, regulates our moods, alters our interactions, and determines our health to such an extent that we barely know ourselves apart from its influence. Sleep lifts and carries our days like water holding lily pads afloat. It takes us out of ourselves in deep, dreamless sleep and poses different viewpoints in our dreams, dislodging us from our fixed ways, opening future possibilities. When we lose sleep or rush in and out of it without looking back, we bind ourselves to the blindness it seeks to remedy.

Sometimes I wonder what we would be like if we truly walked with a foot in both worlds, attending as much to the ambiguities and undoings of sleep as the doings and certainties of waking life. Would we take ourselves so seriously, be so certain we are right, be so willing to give our lives for the causes of others? Maybe, maybe not; but I would like to find out.

ACKNOWLEDGMENTS

This book would never have come into being without the encouragement of my dear friend Debra Schultz, who made me promise to write six hours a week even though I was working full time. Thank you, Debra, for challenging my excuses.

I have been privileged to explore the wonder and mystery of dreams for nearly thirty years with members of my dream group and our mentors, Larry and Pat Sargent. Many fellow writers helped me bring my "sleep project" to fruition. Summer Wood read an early draft out of the kindness of her heart and pointed the way forward. Nancy Ryan, Carol Terry, Jeannie Winer, and Arifa Goodman generously read and discussed early chapters, helping me to clarify my ideas and their expression. Writers at the 2011 A Room of Her Own retreat responded enthusiastically to my reading, and Kate Gale took the time to listen to my pitch, read the opening chapters, and pass my book on to an agent. I am grateful to the founding mothers and attendees of the A Room of Her Own retreat for fostering such an inspiring and supportive writing community for women.

My agent, Elise Capron, has been a constant cheerful champion, keeping the faith when I was flagging, persisting until she found the perfect publisher. Emily Han, my editor at Beyond Words Publishing, shepherded the manuscript toward publication with grace, organization, and vision, and my developmental editor, Sylvia Spratt, helped me to clarify my writing with respectful suggestions along the way. It has been an honor and pleasure to work with so many dedicated professionals in the publishing world.

My biggest thanks and deepest appreciation go to my partner, Kathleen Brennan, whose creative drive continually inspires me and whose faith and generosity in feeding and supporting me while I disappeared to write night after night made this book possible.

NOTES

Prologue

1. Corine Lacrampe, *Sleep and Rest in Animals* (Toronto: Firefly, 2003).
2. Eugene Aserinsky, "The Discovery of REM Sleep," *Journal of the History of the Neurosciences* 5, no. 3 (1996): 213–27, http://www.ncbi.nlm.nih.gov/pubmed/11618742.
3. "Sleep Aids and Insomnia," National Sleep Foundation, accessed April 14, 2013, http://www.sleepfoundation.org/article/sleep-related-problems/sleep-aids-and-insomnia.
4. Laura Barton, "Sleeping Pills: Britain's Hidden Addiction," *Guardian*, August 20, 2012, http://www.theguardian.com/lifeandstyle/2012/aug/20/sleeping-pills-britains-hidden-addiction.
5. "What Are the Most Commonly Traded Commodities?" Investor Guide, January 25, 2013, http://www.investorguide.com/article/11836/what-are-the-most-commonly-traded-commodities-igu/.

Chapter 1—When the Sandman Comes: Falling Asleep

1. Harold Courlander and George Herzog, "The One You Don't See Coming," *The Cow-Tail Switch: And Other West African Stories*, (New York: Henry Holt, 1947): 31–40.
2. J. J. Kockelmans, ed., *Phenomenological Psychology: The Dutch School* (New York: Springer, 1987): 80.

3. C. B. Saper, T. C. Chou, T. E. Scammell, "The Sleep Switch: Hypothalamic Control of Sleep and Wakefulness," *Trends in Neurosciences* 24, no. 12 (2001): 726–31, http://www.ncbi.nlm.nih.gov/pubmed/11718878.
4. Oliver Sacks, "A Neurologist's Notebook: Speed," *New Yorker*, August 23, 2004, http://www.newyorker.com/archive/2004/08/23/040823fa_fact_sacks.
5. Deirdre Barrett, *The Committee of Sleep: How Artists, Scientists, and Athletes Use Dreams for Creative Problem-Solving—and How You Can Too* (New York: Crown, 2001).
6. Herbert Silberer, "Report on a Method of Eliciting and Observing Certain Symbolic Hallucination-Phenomena," in *Organization and Pathology of Thought*, ed. D. Rapaport (New York: Columbia University Press, 1951), 195–207.
7. Gary Lachman, "Hypnagogia," *Fortean Times*, October 2002, http://www.forteantimes.com/features/articles/227/hypnagogia.html.
8. Jean-Luc Nancy, *The Fall of Sleep*, trans. Charlotte Mandell (New York: Fordham University Press, 2009), 7.

Chapter 2—Opening the Inn for Phantoms: Surrendering to Sleep

1. Shelley R. Adler, *Sleep Paralysis: Night-Mares, Nocebos and the Mind-Body Connection* (New Brunswick, NJ: Rutgers University Press, 2011), 15, 100.
2. David J. Hufford, "Sleep Paralysis" interview, *Your Worst Nightmare—Supernatural Assault*, Soul Smack (January 24, 2009), http://www.youtube.com/watch?v=YDp A0MJx780.
3. David J. Hufford, *The Terror That Comes in the Night: An Experience-Centered Study of Supernatural Assault Traditions* (Philadelphia: University of Pennsylvania Press, 1982).
4. J. A. Cheyne, S. D. Rueffer, I. R. Newby-Clark, "Hypnagogic and Hypnopompic Hallucinations During Sleep Paralysis: Neurological and Cultural Construction of the Night-Mare, *Consciousness and Cognition* 8, no. 3 (1999): 333, http://www.ncbi.nlm.nih.gov/pubmed/10487786.
5. Hufford, *Supernatural Assault.*
6. Patrick McNamara, "Sleep Paralysis: When You Wake Up but Can't Move!" *Psychology Today* (December 21, 2011), http://www.psychologytoday.com/blog/dream-catcher/201112/sleep-paralysis.
7. Shahar Arzy, et al., "Induction of an Illusory Shadow Person," *Nature* 443, no. 287 (2006): 287, http://www.nature.com/nature/journal/v443/n7109/abs/443287a.html.

8. Ryan Hurd, "Guarding the Threshold: The Use of Amulets and Liminal Objects for Sleep-Paralysis Nightmares," *Dream Studies* (November 30, 2012), http://dreamstudies.org/2012/11/30/guarding-the-threshold-the-use-of-amulets-and-liminal-objects-for-sleep-paralysis-night-mares/.
9. "Microsleep: Brain Regions Can Take Short Naps During Wakefulness Leading to Errors," *Science Daily*, April 28, 2011, http://www.sciencedaily.com/releases/2011/04/110427131814.htm.
10. Jacob Spilman and Rabbi Menahem Zvi Fischer, "Sleep is 1/60th of Death," accessed April 12, 2013, http://jacobspilman.wordpress.com/2010/12/26/sleep-is-160th-of-death/.
11. William and Marielle Segal, "Sleep and the Inner Landscape," *Parabola 7*, no. 1 (January 1982), 25–38.
12. Yeshi Dhonden, "Sleep and the Inner Landscape," *Parabola* 7, no. 1 (January 1982): 27.
13. Thomas Nelson, *Bedtime Prayers for the Family* (Nashville: Thomas Nelson, 2005), 115.
14. Ira Glass, "Fear of Sleep," *WBEZ Chicago's This American Life*, Episode 361, Aug. 8, 2008, http://www.thisamericanlife.org/radio-archives/episode/361/fear-of-sleep.
15. Occupational Safety and Health Service of the Department of Labour, "Stress and Fatigue: Their Impact on Health and Safety in the Workplace," January 1998, http://www.business.govt.nz/healthandsafetygroup/information-guidance/all-guidance-items/stress-and-fatigue-their-impact-on-health-and-safety-in-the-workplace/stress.pdf.
16. Carol M. Worthman and Melissa K. Melby, "Toward a Comparative Developmental Ecology of Human Sleep," in *Adolescent Sleep Patterns: Biological, Social and Psychological Influences*, ed. Mary A. Carskadon (Cambridge: Cambridge University Press, 2002): 69–117, http://ebooks.cambridge.org/chapter.jsf?bid=CBO9780511499999&cid=CBO9780511499999A014.
17. Gilda A. Morelli et al., "Cultural Variation in Infants' Sleeping Arrangements: Questions of Independence," *Developmental Psychology* 28, no. 4 (1992), http://www.psy.miami.edu/faculty/dmessinger/c_c/rsrcs/rdgs/emot/morelli%20cosleep.dp92.pdf.
18. "Modeh Ani—A Morning Prayer," Jewish Prayers for All Occasions, accessed April 12, 2013, http://www.godweb.org/PrayersJewish.htm.
19. Robert Sack, "Normal Sleep," *Open Spaces: Views form the Northwest* 5, no. 1, accessed April 18, 2013, http://www.open-spaces.com/article-v4n4-sack.php.

Chapter 3—Cribs, Cradles, and Slings: Sleeping Babies Across Cultures

1. O. G. Jenni and B. B. O'Connor, "Children's Sleep: An Interplay between Culture and Biology," *Pediatrics* 115, no. 1 (January 2005): 204–16, http://www.ncbi.nlm.nih.gov/pubmed/15866854; James J. McKenna, "Cultural Influences on Infant and Childhood Sleep Biology, and the Science that Studies It: Toward a More Inclusive Paradigm," in *Sleep and Breathing in Children: A Developmental Approach*, eds. J. Loughlin, J. Carroll, and C. Marcus (Berks, UK: Marcell Dekker, 2000), 199–230; Carol M. Worthman and Melissa K. Melby, "Toward a Comparative Developmental Ecology of Human Sleep;" Mary A. Carskadon, ed., *Sleep Patterns: Biological, Social, and Psychological Influences* (Cambridge: Cambridge University Press, 2002), 69–117.
2. Worthman and Melby, "Toward a Comparative Developmental Ecology of Human Sleep."
3. "Sleeping Disorder Statistics," *Statistic Brain*, February 7, 2013, www.statisticbrain.com/sleeping-disorder-statistics.
4. A. Roger Ekirch, *At Day's Close: Night in Times Past* (New York: W. W. Norton, 2005).
5. Kathleen Pickering, "Decolonizing Time Regimes: Lakota Conceptions of Work, Economy, and Society," *American Anthropologist* 106, no. 1 (2004): 85–97.
6. H. L Ball, "Night-Time Infant Care: Cultural Practice, Evolution and Infant Development," *Child-Rearing and Infant Care Issues: A Cross-Cultural Perspective*, ed. Pranee Liamputtang (Australia: Nova, 2006): 47–61, http://dro.dur.ac.uk/5108/1/5108.pdf.
7. Todd Atteberry, "Daily Life of the American Colonies: The Role of the Tavern in Society," accessed April 12, 2013, http://www.thehistorytrekker.com/daily-life-in-history/daily-life-of-the-american-colonies-the-role-of-the-tavern-in-society.
8. F. F. Schacter et al., "Cosleeping and Sleep Problems in Hispanic-American Urban Young Children," *Pediatrics* 84, no. 3 (September 1989): 522–30; B. Lozoff, G. L. Askew, A. W. Wolf, "Cosleeping and Early Childhood Sleep Problems: Effects of Ethnicity and Socioeconomic Status," *Journal of Developmental and Behavioral Pediatrics* 17, no. 1 (February 1996): 9–15, http://www.ncbi.nlm.nih.gov/pubmed/8675715; S. Farooqi, I. J. Perry, D. G. Beevers, "Ethnic Differences in Sleeping Position and Risk of Cot Death," *Lancet* 338 (1991): 1455, http://www.ncbi.nlm.nih.gov/pubmed/1683436.

9. Toon Van Meijl, "Maori Collective Sleeping as Cultural Resistance," Katie Glaskin and Richard Chenhall, eds., *Sleep Around the World: Anthropological Perspectives* (New York: Palgrave MacMillan, 2013), chapter 7.
10. Heather Munro, "Artifact of the Month: A 19th Centery [sic] Wicker Baby Carriage," Western Illinois Museum Monthly Newsletter (August, 2010), http://westernillinoismuseum.org/artifact_month_2010_august.html; Terry Trucco, "Carriage Trade: Classic Handmade Prams Are Rolling Back into Fashion for London's Toddler Elite," *Chicago Tribune* (April 1, 1987), http://articles.chicagotribune.com/1987-04-01/entertainment/8701250112_1_carriage-trade-restored-high-fashion.
11. Deborah Blum, *Love at Goon Park: Harry Harlow and the Science of Affection* (New York: Basic, 2011); Emily E. Stevens, Thelma E. Patrick, and Rita Pickler, "A History of Infant Feeding," *Journal of Perinatal Education* 18, no. 2 (Spring 2009): 32–39, http://www.ncbi.nlm.nih.gov/pmc/articles/PMC2684040/.
12. Meredith F. Small, *Our Babies, Ourselves: How Biology and Culture Shape the Way We Parent* (New York: Anchor, 1998), 123; D.W. Winnicott, "Transitional Objects and Transitional Phenomena," *Playing and Reality* (London: Tavistock Publications, 1971), 1–18; American Academy of Pediatrics, "Transitional Objects," *Healthy Children*, August 7, 2013, www.healthychildren.org/Englsh/ages-stages/baby/pages/Transitional-Objects.aspx.
13. K. Lee, "The Crying Patterns of Korean Infants and Related Factors," *Developmental Medicine and Child Neurology* 36, no. 7 (1994): 601–7, http://www.ncbi.nlm.nih.gov/pubmed/8034122.
14. Ball, "Night-Time Infant Care."
15. "Babylonian Lullaby: Little Baby in the Dark House," trans. Richard Dumbrill, *BBC World Service*, January 18, 2013, http://www.bbc.co.uk/news/magazine-21041401.
16. Eugene Field, "Wynken, Blynken, and Nod," March 26, 2012, http://www.guardian.co.uk/books/booksblog/2012/mar/26/poem-week-wynken-blynken-nod.
17. Lullabies from the Cradle website, "Mother's Song to Little Hans," *Languages from the Cradle*, 2008, http://lullabies-of-europe.org/UK/DKLullabies/UKDKlullabies.htm.
18. Nancy Shute, "Why Hammocks Make Sleep Easier, Deeper," National Public Radio, June 20, 2011, http://www.npr.org/blogs/health/2011/06/21/137300311/why-hammocks-make-sleep-easier-deeper.

19. "Hammocks' Rocking History," *History in the Headlines*, June 20, 2011, http://www.history.com/news/hammocks-rocking-history.
20. Wanaporn Anuntaseree et al., "Night Waking in Thai Infants at 3 Months of Age: Association between Parental Practices and Infant Sleep," *Sleep Medicine* 9, no. 5 (2008): 564–71, http://www.sciencedirect.com/science/article/pii/S1389945707002663.
21. Antje Richter, "Sleeping Time in Early Chinese Literature," in *Night-Time and Sleep in Asia and the West: Exploring the Dark Side of Life*, eds. Brigitte Steger and Brunt Lodewijk (London: Routledge, 2003), 25.
22. "Babylonian Lullaby: Little Baby in the Dark House;" *BBC News Magazine*, January 18, 2013, www.bbc.co.uk/news/magazine-21041401.
23. Richard Ferber, *Solve Your Child's Sleep Problems: New, Revised and Expanded* (New York: Touchstone, 2006).
24. Barbara Nicholson and Lysa Parker, *Attached at the Heart: Eight Proven Parenting Principles for Raising Connected and Compassionate Children* (Deerfield Beach, FL: Health Communications, 2013).
25. Nils Bergman, "Restoring the Original Paradigm for Infant Care," last updated January 27, 2005, http://www.skin.kangaroomothercare.com/prevtalk01.htm.
26. Jean Liedloff, *The Continuum Concept: In Search of Happiness Lost* (Cambridge: Da Capo, 1986), 49–50.
27. Jaak Panksepp, *Affective Neuroscience: The Foundation of Human and Animal Emotions* (Oxford: Oxford University Press, 2004).
28. W. Middlemiss, D. A. Granger, W. A. Goldberg, L. Nathans, "Asynchrony of Mother-Infant Hypothalamic-Pituitary-Adrenal Axis Activity Following Extinction of Infant Crying Responses Induced During the Transition to Sleep," *Early Human Development* 88, no. 4 (2012): 227–32, http://www.ncbi.nlm.nih.gov/pubmed/21945361.
29. Morelli et al., "Cultural Variation in Infants' Sleeping Arrangements."
30. James J. McKenna, "Cosleeping and Biological Imperatives: Why Human Babies Do Not and Should Not Sleep Alone," *Neuroanthropology*, December 21, 2008, http://neuroanthropology.net/2008/12/21/cosleeping-and-biological-imperatives-why-human-babies-do-not-and-should-not-sleep-alone/.
31. Regine A. Schön and Maarit Silvén, "Natural Parenting—Back to the Basics in Infant Care," *Evolutionary Psychology* 5, no. 1 (2007): 102–83, http://www.epjournal.net/wp-content/uploads/ep05102183.pdf.
32. Daniel J. Siegel, *The Developing Mind: How Relationships and the Brain Interact to Shape Who We Are*, 2nd ed. (London: Guilford, 2012).

33. J. P. Henry and S. Wang, "Effects of Early Stress on Adult Affiliative Behavior," *Psychoneuroendocrinology* 23, no. 8 (1998): 836–75; Schön and Silvén, "Natural Parenting—Back to the Basics in Infant Care."
34. M. R. Gunnar and B. Donzella, "Social Regulation of the Cortisol Levels in Early Human Development," *Psychoneuroendocrinology* 27, no. 1–2 (2002): 199–220, http://www.ncbi.nlm.nih.gov/pubmed/11750779.
35. J. Mosenkis, "The Effects of Childhood Cosleeping on Later Life Development" (master's thesis, Department of Human Development, University of Chicago, Chicago, IL, 1998); J. F. Forbes, D. S. Weiss, R. A. Folen, "The Cosleeping Habits of Military Children," *Military Medicine* 157, no. 4 (1992): 196–200, http://www.ncbi.nlm.nih.gov/pubmed/1620382; C. Joanne Crawford, "Parenting Practices in the Basque Country: Implications of Infant and Childhood Sleeping Location for Personality Development," *Ethos* 22, no. 1 (1994): 42–82, http://www.jstor.org/discover/10.2307/640468?uid=3739816&uid=2&uid=4&uid=3739256&sid=21102033182991; B. Hewlett, M. Lamb, *Hunter-Gatherer Childhoods: Evolutionary, Developmental, and Cultural Perspectives* (Piscataway, NJ: Transaction, 2005).

Chapter 4—Sleep Stages: Western Science and Eastern Philosophy

1. Tina Hesman Saey, "The Why of Sleep," *Science News* 17 (October 24, 2009), http://www.sciencenews.org/pictures/sleep/sn_sleep_fulledition_lo.pdf.
2. J. A. Hobson, "REM Sleep and Dreaming: Towards a Theory of Protoconsciousness," *Nature Reviews, Neuroscience* 10, no. 11 (Nov 2009): 803–13, http://www.ncbi.nlm.nih.gov/pubmed/19794431.
3. Benedict Carey, "A Dream Interpretation: Tuneups for the Brain," *New York Times* (November 9, 2009), http://www.nytimes.com/2009/11/10/health/10mind.html.
4. Oliver Sacks, *An Anthropologist on Mars* (New York: Vintage, 1996), 153–87.
5. Marcus E. Raichle and Abraham Z. Snyder, "A Default Mode of Brain Function: A Brief History of an Evolving Idea," *NeuroImage* (2007), http://139.127.252.17/bijclub/20070504/raichle07.pdf; Kelly Crowe, "Seeking Seat of Consciousness in Dark Side of Brain," CBC News, January 3, 2013, http://www.sott.net/article/255694-Seeking-seat-of-consciousness-in-dark-side-of-brain.

6. Virginia Woolf, *Mrs. Dalloway* (New York: Harcourt Brace Jovanovich, 1925), 99.
7. "August Strindberg: 'I'm a Devilish Fellow Who Can Do Many Tricks,'" (Stockholm: The Swedish Institute, 2012), http://www.sweden.se/eng/Home/Lifestyle/Literature/Facts/August-Strindberg/.
8. Robert Sapolsky, "Wild Dreams," *Discover Magazine*, April 1, 2001, http://discovermagazine.com/2001/apr/cover#.UWtbx7U4uHg.
9. Lawrence P. Riso et al., *Cognitive Schemas and Core Beliefs in Psychological Problems: A Scientist-Practitioner Guide* (Washington, DC: American Psychological Association, 2007).
10. Antti Revonsuo, "The Reinterpretation of Dreams: An Evolutionary Hypothesis of the Function of Dreaming," *Behavioral and Brain Sciences* 23 (2000): 793–1121, http://www.ncbi.nlm.nih.gov/pubmed/11515147; K. Valli et al., "The Threat Stimulation Theory of the Evolutionary Function of Dreaming: Evidence from Dreams of Traumatized Children," *Consciousness and Cognition* 14, no. 1 (March 2005): 188–218, http://www.ncbi.nlm.nih.gov/pubmed/15766897; Jay Dixit, "Dreams: Night School," *Psychology Today*, November 1, 2007, http://www.psychologytoday.com/articles/200710/dreams-night-school.
11. Patrick McNamara, *An Evolutionary Psychology of Sleep and Dreams* (Westport, CT: Praeger, 2004); Patrick McNamara, "Counterfactual Thoughts in Dreams," *Dreaming* 10, no. 4 (2000): 237–46.
12. Marcos G. Frank, Naoum P. Issa, Michael P. Styker, "Sleep Enhances Plasticity in the Developing Visual Cortex," *Neuron* 30 (April 2001): 275–87, http://www.cscb.northwestern.edu/jcpdfs/frank01.pdf.
13. Carl Sagan, *The Dragons of Eden: Speculations on the Evolution of Human Intelligence* (New York: Ballantine, 1986), 146, 158.
14. David Foulkes, *Children's Dreaming and the Evolution of Consciousness* (Cambridge, MA: Harvard University Press, 1999), 60–65.
15. Silvina G. Horovitz et al., "Decoupling of the Brain's Default Mode Network During Deep Sleep," *Proceedings of the National Academy of Sciences* 106, no. 27 (July 7, 2009): 11376–81, http://www.ncbi.nlm.nih.gov/pmc/articles/PMC2708777/.
16. Benedict Carey, "Aging in Brain Found to Hurt Sleep Needed for Memory," *New York Times*, January 27, 2013, http://www.nytimes.com/2013/01/28/health/brain-aging-linked-to-sleep-related-memory-decline.html?ref=benedictcarey.
17. Huston Smith, Swami Satprakashananda, Methods of Knowledge *Perceptual, Nonperceptual and Transcendental According to the Advaita*

Vedanta (London: Allen & Unwin, 1965), forward.
18. V. Jayaram, trans., *The Mandukya Upanishad*, Hindu Website, accessed April 18, 2013, http://www.hinduwebsite.com/mandukya.asp.
19. Arvind Sharma, *Sleep as a State of Consciousness in Advaita Vedanta* (Albany: State University of New York Press, 2004).
20. Zara Houshmand, Robert B. Livingston, and B. Alan Wallace, eds., *Consciousness at the Crossroads: Conversations with the Dalai Lama on Brain Science and Buddhism* (Boston: Snow Lion, 1999); Richard King, *Early Advaita Vedanta and Buddhism: The Mahayana Context of the Guadapadiya-Kārika* (Albany: State University of New York Press, 1995).
21. Hazrat Inayat Kahn, "The Mystery of Sleep," *The Art of Being*, vol. VIII, *Health and Order of Body and Mind*, accessed April 18, 2013, http://wahiduddin.net/mv2/VIII/VIII_1_21.htm.
22. Mewlana Jalaluddin Rumi, F. Hadland Davis, trans., "Sleep of the Body the Soul's Awakening" (1912), http://www.poemhunter.com/poem/sleep-of-the-body-the-soul-s-awakening/.
23. Richard Miller, *Yoga Nidra: A Meditative Practice for Deep Relaxation and Healing* (Boulder, CO: Sounds True, 2005).
24. Juan Li, "Playing with the Clouds: The Foundations of Taoist Dream Yoga," Artikel, accessed April 13, 2013, http://www.healingtao.org/deutsch/artikel2.htm; Peter Ochiogrosso, "Dream Yoga," *Yoga Journal* (January/February 1997), http://www.natural-connection.com/resource/yoga_journal/dream_yoga.html.

Chapter 5—Between Sleeps: The Midnight Watch

1. T. A. Wehr, "In Short Photoperiods, Human Sleep is Biphasic," *Journal of Sleep Research* 1, no. 2 (June 1992): 103–7; Verlyn Klinkenborg, "Awakening to Sleep," *New York Times Magazine*, January 5, 1997, http://www.nytimes.com/1997/01/05/magazine/awakening-to-sleep.html?pagewanted=all&src=pm; Natalie Angier, "Modern Life Suppresses an Ancient Body Rhythm, *New York Times*, March 14, 1995, http://www.nytimes.com/1995/03/14/science/modern-life-suppresses-an-ancient-body-rhythm.html?scp=6&sq=dr%20thomas%20wehr&st=cse&pagewanted=all.
2. A. Roger Ekirch, *At Day's Close: Night in Times Past* (New York: W. W. Norton, 2005), 300–302.
3. E. B. Cowell, trans., *The Buddha-Carita of Ásvaghosa*, vol. XIV, *Enlightenment*, accessed April 14, 2013, http://www.buddhanet-de.net/

ancient-buddhist-texts/English-Texts/Buddhacarita/14-Book-XIV.htm.

4. Mark Pendergrast, *Uncommon Grounds: The History of Coffee and How It Transformed our World* (New York: Basic, 2010), 16–18; Mathew Green, "London Cafes: The Surprising History of London's Lost Coffeehouses," *The Telegraph* (March 20, 2012).
5. "2008 Sleep, Performance and the Workplace," National Sleep Foundation, accessed April 28, 2013, http://www.sleepfoundation.org/article/sleep-america-polls/2008-sleep-performance-and-the-workplace.
6. Thomas A. Wehr. "The Impact of Changes in Nightlength (Scotoperiod) on Human Sleep," in: *Regulation of Sleep and Circadian Rhythms*, eds., F. W. Turek and P. C. Zee (New York: Marcel Dekker; 1999), 263-285, http://www.psychiatrictimes.com/sleep-disorders/acknowledging-preindustrial-patterns-sleep-may-revolutionize-approach-sleep-dysfunction#sthash.YBlqzikD.dpuf.
7. Robert Roy Britt, "Sleep Deprived? You May Need Less as You Age," NBC News, last updated February 1, 2010, http://www.nbcnews.com/id/35180414/ns/healthaging/t/sleep-deprived-you-may-need-less-you-age/%20-%20.UX2vL7U4uHg#UlWsJhbnbl0.
8. Blake Butler, *Nothing: A Portrait of Insomnia* (New York: HarperCollins, 2011).
9. Walter A. Brown, "Broken Sleep May Be Natural Sleep," *Psychiatric Times* (March 1, 2007), http://www.psychiatrictimes.com/articles/broken-sleep-may-be-natural-sleep.
10. Lisa Russ Spaar, "Insomnia and the Poet," *New York Times*, March 9, 2013, http://opinionator.blogs.nytimes.com/2013/03/09/insomnia-and-the-poet/.

Chapter 6—When Sleep Never Comes: Insomnia's Toll

1. Hannah Morphy et al., "Epidemiology of Insomnia: A Longitudinal Study in a UK Population," *Sleep* 30, no. 3, (2007): 274–280, http://www.ncbi.nlm.nih.gov/pubmed/17425223.
2. Wen-siang, Thomas Cleary, trans., *Sleepless Nights: Verses for the Wakeful* (Berkeley: North Atlantic, 1995), 70.
3. Sahoo Saddicha, "Diagnosis and Treatment of Chronic Insomnia," *Annals of Indian Academy of Neurology* 13, no. 2 (April–June 2010): 94–102.
4. "Americans Crave Sleep More Than Sex, Says Better Sleep Council Survey," Better Sleep Council, April 30, 2012, http://bettersleep.org/press-room/press-releases/americans-crave-sleep-more-than-sex-says-

better-sleep-council-survey.

5. Sean Coughlan, "Lack of Sleep Blights Pupils' Education," BBC News, May 8, 2013, http://www.bbc.co.uk/news/business-22209818.
6. "Workplace stress steals an hour and a quarter of our sleep every night," September 5, 2013, http://www.travelodge.co.uk/press_releases/press_release.php?id=524.
7. Charles A. Czeisler, "Perspective: Casting Light on Sleep Deficiency," *Nature* 497 (May 23, 2013), http://www.nature.com/nature/journal/v497/n7450_supp/full/497S13a.html.
8. C. Cajochen et al., "Evening Exposure to Light-Emitting Diodes (LED)-Backlit Computer Screen Affects Circadian Physiology and Cognitive Performance," *Journal of Applied Physiology* 110, no. 5 (May 2011): 1432–8, http://www.ncbi.nlm.nih.gov/pubmed/21415172.
9. T. W. Boonstra et al., "Effects of Sleep Deprivation on Neural Functioning: An Integrative Review," *Cellular and Molecular Life Sciences* 64, no. 7–8 (April 2007): 935–46, http://www.ncbi.nlm.nih.gov/pmc/articles/PMC2778638/; Bronwyn Fryer, "Sleep Deficit: The Performance Killer, A Conversation with Charles A. Czeisler," *Harvard Business Review* (October 2006), http://hbr.org/2006/10/sleep-deficit-the-performance-killer.
10. Léger et al., "An International Survey of Sleeping Problems."
11. "Sleep and Sleep Disorders," Centers for Disease Control and Prevention, last updated March 14, 2013, http://www.cdc.gov/features/sleep/.
12. Vistal G. Thakkar, "Diagnosing the Wrong Deficit," *New York Times*, April 27, 2013, Sunday Review, http://www.nytimes.com/2013/04/28/opinion/sunday/diagnosing-the-wrong-deficit.html?_r=0.
13. Karine Spiegel, Rachel Leproult, and Eve Van Cauter, "Impact of Sleep Debt on Metabolic and Endocrine Function," *Lancet*, 354, no. 9188 (October 23, 1999): 1435–9, http://www.sciencedirect.com/science/article/pii/S0140673699013768.
14. Karine Spiegel et al., "Brief Communication: Sleep Curtailment in Healthy Young Men Is Associated with Decreased Leptin Levels, Elevated Ghrelin Levels, and Increased Hunger and Appetite," *Annals of Internal Medicine* 141, no. 11 (December 2004): 846–51, http://isites.harvard.edu/fs/docs/icb.topic197607.files/Due_Wk_11_Nov_28/SPIEGEL_2004.pdf.
15. "Sleep and Sleep Disorders," Centers for Disease Control and Prevention.
16. C. Hublin et al., "Sleep and Mortality: A Population-Based 22-Year Follow-Up Study," *Sleep* 30, no. 10 (2007): 1245–53, http://www.ncbi.nlm.nih.gov/pubmed/17969458.

17. C. S. Fichten, "Long Sleepers Sleep More and Short Sleepers Sleep Less: A Comparison of Older Adults Who Sleep Well," *Behavioral Sleep Medicine* 2, no. 1 (2004): 2–23, http://www.ncbi.nlm.nih.gov/pubmed/15600221.
18. Patrick Levy and Wilfred Pigeon, "Sleep Disorders Associated with Decreased Slow-Wave Sleep," in *Slow-Wave Sleep: Beyond Insomnia: The Importance of Slow-Wave Sleep for Your Patients*, ed. Dijk Derk-Jan et al. (London: Wolters Kluwer Health Pharma Solutions, 2010), 117–32.
19. A. Nehliq, J. L. Daval, G. Debry, "Caffeine and the Central Nervous System: Mechanisms of Action, Biochemical, Metabolic and Psychostimulant Effects," *Brain Research Reviews* 17, no. 2 (May–August 1992): 139–70, http://www.ncbi.nlm.nih.gov/pubmed/1356551.
20. Ray Gustini, "95% of People Who Say they Need Five Hours of Sleep Are Wrong," *Atlantic Wire*, April 5, 2011, http://www.theatlanticwire.com/national/2011/04/95-percent-people-who-say-they-need-five-hours-sleep-are-wrong/36366/.
21. Interview with Bill Clinton by Wolf Blitzer, *The Situation Room*, CNN, December 3, 2008, http://transcripts.cnn.com/TRANSCRIPTS/0812/03/sitroom.03.html.
22. A. Williamson and A. Feyer, "Moderate Sleep Deprivation Produces Impairments in Cognitive and Motor Performance Equivalent to Legally Prescribed Levels of Alcohol Intoxication," *Occupational and Environmental Medicine* 57, no. 10 (October 2000): 649–55, http://www.ncbi.nlm.nih.gov/pmc/articles/PMC1739867/; Hans P. A. Van Dongen et al., "The Cumulative Cost of Additional Wakefulness: Dose-Response Effects on Neurobehavioral Functions and Sleep Physiology from Chronic Sleep Restriction and Total Sleep Deprivation" *Sleep* 26, no. 2 (2003): 117–26, http://www.med.upenn.edu/uep/user_documents/dfd16.pdf.
23. See note 6.
24. Craig Lambert, "Deep into Sleep," *Harvard Magazine*, July–August 2005, http://harvardmagazine.com/2005/07/deep-into-sleep.html.
25. Mary Jo De Lonardo, "Go to Bed! Getting Teens to Get Enough Sleep," WebMD (October 4, 2012), www.webmd.com/parenting/raising-fit-kids/recharge/help-teens-get-sleep; Till Roenneberg, *Internal Time: Chronotypes, Social Jet Lag, and Why You're So Tired* (Cambridge, MA: Harvard University Press, 2012); Mary Carskadon, ed., *Adolescent Sleep Patterns: Biological, Social, and Psychological Influences* (Cambridge: Cambridge University Press, 2002), 96–113.
26. H. R. Colton and B. M. Altevogt, eds., *Sleep Disorders and Sleep*

Deprivation (Washington, DC: National Academic Press, 2006), http://www.ncbi.nlm.nih.gov/books/NBK19961/.

27. Jane E. Brody, "Cheating Ourselves of Sleep," *New York Times* (June 17, 2013), http://well.blogs.nytimes.com/2013/06/17/cheating-ourselves-of-sleep/?_r=0.
28. Stanford Center for Sleep Sciences, "Exploring New Frontiers in Human Health," *The Stanford Challenge*, accessed April 27, 2013, http://neuroscience.stanford.edu/research/programs/program_info/Sleep%20Science_011609B_compress.pdf.
29. Jim Horne, "Insomnia: Good Night, and Good Luck," *Telegraph*, March 4, 2008, http://www.telegraph.co.uk/science/science-news/3334782/Insomnia-Good-night-and-good-luck.html.
30. Bonnie Rochman, "A History of Kids and Sleep: Why They Never Get Enough," *Time*, February 13, 2012, http://healthland.time.com/2012/02/13/a-history-of-kids-and-sleep-its-never-enough/.
31. Centers for Disease Control, "Perceived Insufficient Rest or Sleep Among Adults—United States, 2008," *Morbidity and Mortality Weekly Report*, October 30, 2009, http://www.cdc.gov/mmwr/preview/mmwrhtml/mm5842a2.htm.
32. Horne, "Insomnia: Good Night, and Good Luck."
33. American Academy of Sleep Medicine, "Study Links Workplace Daylight Exposure to Sleep, Activity and Quality of Life," American Academy of Sleep Medicine Press Release (June 7, 2013), http://www.aasmnet.org/articles.aspx?id=3943.
34. Worthman and Melby, "Toward a Comparative Developmental Ecology of Human Sleep."
35. Charles Q. Choi, "(Dis)United States of Sleep: U.S.-Born Americans' Sleep Patterns Differ from Those of Immigrants," *Scientific American*, June 18, 2012, http://www.scientificamerican.com/article.cfm?id=us-born-americans-sleep-patterns-dffer-from-immigrants.
36. Maria Basta et al., "Chronic Insomnia and Stress System," *Sleep Medicine Clinics Journal* 2, no. 2 (2007): 279–91.
37. "Meditation May Be an Effective Treatment for Insomnia," *Science Daily*, June 15, 2009, http://www.sciencedaily.com/releases/2009/06/090609072719.htm; Michael J. Breus, "Yoga Can Help with Insomnia," *Huffington Post*, October 20, 2012, http://www.huffingtonpost.com/dr-michael-j-breus/yoga-insomnia_b_1939696.html; P. J. Hauri et al, "The Treatment of Psychophysiologic Insomnia with Biofeedback: A Replication Study," *Biofeedback and Self-Regulation* 7, no. 2 (June 1982): 223–35, http://www.

ncbi.nlm.nih.gov/pubmed/7138954; K. Hoedlmoser et al., "Instrumental Conditioning of Human Sensorimotor Rhythm (12–15 Hz) and its Impact on Sleep as Well as Declarative Learning," *Sleep* 31, no. 10 (2008): 1401–8.

Chapter 7—Downers, Benzos, and Z-Drugs: The Commercialization of Sleep

1. Andrea Tone, *The Age of Anxiety: A History of America's Turbulent Affair with Tranquilizers* (New York: Basic, 2008), 21; Sarena Fuller, "The History of Sleep Aids," eHow, accessed April 20, 2013, http://www.ehow.com/about_5130860_history-sleep-aids.html.
2. "Bromide Sleep," *Merck's Archives*, 1900; 2(3), 110–1, quoted in Howard H. Chiang, "An Early Hope of Psychopharmacology: Bromide Treatment in the Twentieth-Century Psychiatry," *Historia Medicinæ* 1, no. 1 (April 20, 2009), http://www.medicinae.org/e06.
3. Tone, *The Age of Anxiety*, 69–116.
4. Tone, *The Age of Anxiety*, 1–26; Edward Shorter, *A History of Psychiatry: From the Era of the Asylum to the Age of Prozac* (New York: Wiley and Sons, 1997), 69–145; Francisco López-Muñoz et al., "The History of Barbiturates a Century after Their Clinical Introduction," *Journal of Neuropsychiatric Disease and Treatment* 1, no. 4 (December, 2005): 329–43, http://www.ncbi.nlm.nih.gov/pmc/articles/PMC2424120/.
5. Bara Fintel et al., "The Thalidomide Tragedy: Lessons for Drug Safety and Regulation," *Science in Society*, July 28, 2009, http://scienceinsociety.northwestern.edu/content/articles/2009/research-digest/thalidomide/title-tba; Russell Mokhiber, "The Tragic Children of Thalidomide," *Corporate Crime and Violence* 8, no. 4 (April 1987), http://multinationalmonitor.org/hyper/issues/1987/04/thalidomide.html.
6. Tracy Conner, "JFK Popped Lots of Pills," *New York Daily News*, November 17, 2002, 3.
7. D. F. Kripke, "Chronic Hypnotic Use: Deadly Risks, Doubtful Benefit," *Sleep Medicine Reviews* 4, no. 1 (February 2000): 5–20, http://www.ncbi.nlm.nih.gov/pubmed/12531158.
8. C. Heather Ashton, "Protracted Withdrawal Symptoms from Benzodiazepines," in *Comprehensive Handbook of Drug and Alcohol Addiction*, ed. Norman Miller (New York: Marcel Dekker, 1991), 915–31.
9. Anne Milton, "Prescribed Addiction," *Face the Facts*, BBC Radio, July 27, 2011, http://www.bbc.co.uk/programmes/b012wxxw.
10. D. W. Kaufman et al., "Recent Patterns of Medication Use in the

Ambulatory Adult Population of the United States: The Slone Survey," *Journal of the American Medical Association* 287, no. 3 (January 16, 2002): 337–44.

11. Dani Veracity, "Ambien Sleeping Pills Linked to Bizarre Sleep Walking Behavior, Including Unconscious Driving of Vehicles and Wild Hallucinations," *Natural News*, June 8, 2006, http://www.naturalnews.com/019413_Ambien_drug_side_effects.html.
12. "Bitter Pill Awards 2006: The 'While You Were Sleeping' Award: For Overmarketing Insomnia Medications to Anyone Who's Ever Had a Bad Night's Sleep," *Prescription Access Litigation*, accessed April 20, 2013, http://www.prescriptionaccess.org/learnmore?id=0015.
13. Jerome Burne, "Take Ambien and you'll only get an extra 15 minutes sleep and could be hooked for life," *Daily Mail*, January 28, 2008, http://www.dailymail.co.uk/health/article-510940/Take-Ambien-youll-extra-15-minutes-sleep---hooked-life.html.
14. Stephanie Saul, "Some Sleeping Pill Users Range Far Beyond Bed," *New York Times*, March 8, 2006, http://www.nytimes.com/2006/03/08/business/08ambien.html?pagewanted=all&_r=0.
15. Kai Falkenberg, "While You Were Sleeping," *Marie Claire*, September 27, 2012, http://www.marieclaire.com/world-reports/while-you-were-sleeping#.
16. Ibid.
17. Michelle Castillo, "ER Visits Tied to Ambien, Other Insomnia Drugs up 220% in Recent Years," CBS News, May 1, 2013, http://www.cbsnews.com/8301-204_162-57582345/er-visits-tied-to-ambien-other-insomnia-drugs-up-220-in-recent-years/.
18. Christopher Leibig, "The Ambien Defense: Criminal Law Unclear on How to Treat the 'Ambien Zombie' Phenomenon," *Examiner*, August 29, 2010, http://www.examiner.com/article/the-ambien-defense-criminal-law-unclear-on-how-to-treat-the-ambien-zombie-phenomenon.
19. January W. Payne, "Report: Go Easy on Sleeping Pills," *Washington Post*, August 15, 2006, http://www.washingtonpost.com/wp-dyn/content/article/2006/08/14/AR2006081400875.html.
20. Jerry Siegel, "Are Sleeping Pills Good for You?" *Huffington Post*, February 4, 2010, http://www.huffingtonpost.com/jerry-siegel/are-sleeping-pills-good-f_b_446804.html; Paul Spector, MD, "Sleep on Drugs," *Huffington Post*, September 26, 2012, http://www.huffingtonpost.com/paul-spector-md/sleeping-pills_b_1917116.html.
21. "Bitter Pill Awards 2006."

22. Stephanie Saul, "Sleep Drugs Found Only Mildly Effective, but Wildly Popular," *New York Times*, October 23, 2007, http://www.nytimes.com/2007/10/23/health/23drug.html?pagewanted=all.
23. Andrew Hough, "Benefits of Sleeping Pills 'Come from Placebo Effect,'" *Telegraph*, December 20, 2012, http://www.telegraph.co.uk/health/healthnews/9757450/Benefits-of-sleeping-pills-come-from-placebo-effect.html; Klinkenborg, "Awakening to Sleep." *New York Times Magazine*, January 5, 1997, http://www.nytimes.com/1997/01/05/magazine/awakening-to-sleep.html.
24. Stanley Coren, *Sleep Thieves: An Eye-Opening Exploration into the Science and Mysteries of Sleep* (New York: Simon and Schuster, 1997), 15.
25. Aaron B. Holley and Christopher J. Lettieri, "Sleep in the ICU," *Medscape*, June 23, 2010, http://www.medscape.com/viewarticle/723907; Margarita Tartakovsky, "The First Line of Treatment for Insomnia That'll Surprise You," PsychCentral, 2011, http://psychcentral.com/lib/2011/the-first-line-of-treatment-for-insomnia-thatll-surprise-you/all/1/.
26. "Cognitive Behavioral Therapy for Insomnia," National Sleep Foundation, accessed April 20, 2013, http://www.sleepfoundation.org/article/hot-topics/cognitive-behavioral-therapy-insomnia.
27. Charles M. Morin, "Cognitive-Behavioral Therapy of Insomnia," *Sleep Medicine Clinics* 1 (2006): 375–86. https://wiki.umms.med.umich.edu/download/attachments/125274436/Cognitive+Behavioral+Therapy+of+Insomnia.pdf?version=1&modificationDate=1341006540000.
28. A. N. Vgontzas et al., "Adverse Effects of Modest Sleep Restriction on Sleepiness, Performance, and Inflammatory Cytokines," *Journal of Clinical Endocrinology and Metabolism* 89, no. 5 (May 2004): 2119. http://jcem.endojournals.org/content/89/5/2119.full.
29. J. D. Edinger, "Cognitive Behavioral Therapy for Treatment of Chronic Primary Insomnia: A Randomized Controlled Trial," *Journal of the American Medical Association* 285, no. 14 (April 11, 2001): 1856–64, http://www.ncbi.nlm.nih.gov/pubmed/11308399.
30. Iris Rosendahl, "Sleep Aids: Bright Spot in Sluggish Market," *Drug Topics*, November 23, 1992, http://business.highbeam.com/62489/article-1G1-12990441/sleep-aids-bright-spot-sluggish-market; Michael Myser, "$20 Billion for a Good Night's Rest," *Business 2.0 Magazine*, March 15, 2007, http://money.cnn.com/magazines/business2/business2_archive/2006/10/01/8387112/index.htm.
31. Melanie Wells, "The Sleep Racket: Who's Making Big Bucks off Your

Insomnia?" *Forbes*, February 27, 2006, http://www.forbes.com/forbes/2006/0227/080.html.

32. Elizabeth Large, "Dreaming of Sleep," *Baltimore Sun*, March 1, 2007, http://articles.baltimoresun.com/2007-03-11/news/0703120246_1_sleep-bed-eight-hours.
33. Eve Van Cauter et al., "The Impact of Sleep Deprivation on Hormones and Metabolism," *MedScape Neurology* 7, no. 1 (2005), http://www.medscape.org/viewarticle/502825.
34. John W. Shepard et al., "History of the Development of Sleep Medicine in the United States," *Journal of Clinical Sleep Medicine* 1, no. 1 (January 15, 2005): 61–82, http://www.ncbi.nlm.nih.gov/pmc/articles/PMC2413168/; Dorsey Griffith and Steve Wiegand, "A Little Too Cosy? Not-for-Profits May Have Undisclosed Funding Ties to For-Profit Drug Companies," *Sacramento Bee*, July 13, 2005, http://www.pharmadisclose.org/spgppd/sb050713.html.
35. "Drowsy Driving: Talking Points," National Sleep Foundation, accessed April 20, 2013, http://www.sleepfoundation.org/sites/default/files/Drowsy%20Driving-Key%20Messages%20and%20Talking%20Points.pdf.
36. Luiza Ch. Savage, "Sleep Crisis: The Science of Slumber," *Maclean's*, June 17, 2013, http://www2.macleans.ca/2013/06/17/the-sleep-crisis/.
37. Christian J. Krautkramer, "Language, Print Media, and Medicalization of Sleep Disorders," *American Medical Association Journal of Ethics* 10, no. 9 (September 2008): 564–67, http://virtualmentor.ama-assn.org/2008/09/jdsc1-0809.html; Simon J. Williams, "Sleep and Health: Sociological Reflections on the Dormant Society," *Health: An Interdisciplinary Journal for the Social Study of Health, Illness and Medicine* 6, no. 2 (April 2002), 173–200.
38. "NHS sleeping pill spend leaps to £50m," *Guardian*, May 11, 2012, http://www.theguardian.com/society/2012/may/11/nhs-spending-sleeping-pills-50m.
39. Jennifer Soong, "Living with Insomnia: Get a Good Night's Sleep/Sleeping Pills: Prescription or OTC?" WebMD, last reviewed March 2, 2011, http://www.webmd.com/sleep-disorders/living-with-insomnia-11/sleeping-pills; Rachel Grumman, "When to Take a Sleeping Pill," *CNN Health*, December 9, 2008, http://www.cnn.com/2008/HEALTH/09/19/healthmag.sleeping.pills/index.html?_s=PM:HEALTH.

Chapter 8—The Social Divide: Separating Sleep from Consciousness

1. Varela, *Sleeping, Dreaming, and Dying.*
2. Ibid.
3. Gerald Bullett, "The Other 'I,'" in *The World of Dreams*, ed. R. L. Woods (New York: Random House, 1947), 920.
4. Martin Prechtel, class teaching in Taos, NM, 1990.
5. Richter, "Sleeping Time in Early Chinese Literature."
6. Anthony Shafton, *Dream-Singers: The African-American Way with Dreams* (New York: Wiley & Sons, 2002).
7. Mircea Eliade, "Sleep," *Plural Magazine*, 2007, http://www.icr.ro/bucuresti/identity-and-destiny-ideas-and-ideology-in-interwar-romania-29-2007/sleep.html.
8. Wai-yee Li, "Dreams of Interpretation in Early Chinese Historical and Philosophical Writings," in *Dream Cultures: Explorations in the Comparative History of Dreaming*, eds. David Shulman and Guy G. Stroumsa (New York: Oxford University Press, 1999), 37.
9. Ernest Hartmann, "Boundaries and Dreams," 2006, http://www.tufts.edu/~ehartm01/.
10. Catherine Clément, *Syncope: The Philosophy of Rapture*, trans. Sally O'Driscoll (St. Paul, MN: University of Minnesota Press, 1994).
11. Vladimir Nabokov, *Pale Fire* (New York: Vintage, 1989), 30.
12. Jess Stearn, *Edgar Cayce: The Sleeping Prophet* (New York: Doubleday, 1967).
13. Barbara Tedlock, ed., "Dreaming and Dream Research," *Dreaming: Anthropological and Psychological Interpretations* (Santa Fe: School of American Research Press, 1992), 1–300.

Chapter 9—When Sleeping Birds Fly: Half Awake and Half Asleep

1. Kathleen McAuliffe, "What Breaks Down the Asleep/Awake Divide?" *Discover*, August 10, 2007, http://discovermagazine.com/2007/medical-mysteries/what-breaks-down-the-asleep-awake-divide#.Ug0w5D8luuQ.
2. James M. Krueger et al., "Sleep as a Fundamental Property of Neuronal Assemblies," *Nature Reviews Neuroscience* 9 (2008): 910-19, http://www.nature.com/nrn/journal/v9/n12/abs/nrn2521.html.

3. Cherie Winner, "Sleep Creeps Up: No Top-Down Control for Sleep and Wakefulness, WSU Scientists Find," *Washington State University Research News & Features*, last updated March 4, 2009, http://researchnews.wsu.edu/health/219.html.
4. Chiarra Cirelli and Giulio Tononi, "Is Sleep Essential?" *PLOS Biology* 6, no. 8 (2008), http://www.plosbiology.org/article/info:doi/10.1371/journal.pbio.0060216.
5. C. Rattenborg et al., "Behavioral, Neurophysiological and Evolutionary Perspectives on Unihemispheric Sleep," *Neuroscience and Biobehavioral Reviews* 24, no. 8 (2000): 817–42, http://www.ncbi.nlm.nih.gov/pubmed/11118608.
6. John Lesku et al, "Brain Regions Sleep More Deeply When Used More—Also in Birds," *Phys.Org*, January 12, 2011, http://phys.org/news/2011-01-brain-regions-deeply-birds.htmlews/2011-01-brain-regions-deeply-birds.html; Victor Vladyslav et al., "Local Sleep in Awake Rats," *Nature* 472, no. 7344 (April 28, 2011), http://www.ncbi.nlm.nih.gov/pmc/articles/PMC3085007/.
7. Yuval Nir et al., "Regional Slow Waves and Spindles in Human Sleep," *Neuron* 70, no. 1 (April 14, 2011), 153–169.
8. Oliver Sacks, "Enjoying Getting to Sleep" (video recording), *Web of Stories* 339, accessed April 12, 2013, http://www.webofstories.com/play/54514.
9. John Steinbeck, *Sweet Thursday* (New York, Penguin, 2008), 71.
10. Timothy D. Wilson, *Stranger to Ourselves: Discovering the Adaptive Unconscious* (Cambridge, MA: Harvard University Press, 2002).
11. Rosalind D. Cartwright, *The Twenty-Four Hour Mind: The Role of Sleep and Dreaming in Our Emotional Lives* (New York: Oxford University Press, 2010).

Chapter 10—The Invisible Labors of Sleep: Memory and Invention

1. Rubin Naiman, "Narcolepsy: What We All Should Know," *Huffington Post*, August 7, 2012, http://www.huffingtonpost.com/rubin-naiman-phd/narcolepsy_b_1730627.html.
2. Matthew P. Walker, "The Role of Slow-Wave Sleep in Memory Processing," *Journal of Clinical Sleep Medicine* 5, no. 2 Suppl. (April 15, 2009): S20–S26, http://www.ncbi.nlm.nih.gov/pmc/articles/PMC2824214/.
3. Mathew P. Walker et al., "Practice with Sleep Makes Perfect: Sleep-

Dependent Motor Skill Learning," *Neuron* 35 (July 3, 2002): 205–11, http://walkerlab.berkeley.edu/reprints/Walker%20et%20al._Neuron_2002.pdf; Craig Lambert, "Deep into Sleep," *Harvard Magazine*, July–August 2005, http://harvardmagazine.com/2005/07/deep-into-sleep.html.

4. Nikhil Swaminathan, "Slumber Reruns: As We Sleep, Our Brains Research the Day," *Scientific American*, November 19, 2007, http://www.scientificamerican.com/article.cfm?id=slumber-reruns-as-we-sleep.
5. Giulio Tononi and Chiara Cirelli, "Sleep Function and Synaptic Homeostasis," *Sleep Medicine Reviews* 10 (2006): 49–62, http://isites.harvard.edu/fs/docs/icb.topic1075442.files/Week%207/Tononi%20and%20Cirelli%20-%202006%20-%20Sleep%20function%20and%20synaptic%20homeostasis.pdf
6. M. P. Walker and R. Stickgold, "Sleep, Memory, and Plasticity," *Annual Review of Psychology* 57 (2006): 139–66, http://www.ncbi.nlm.nih.gov/pubmed/16318592.
7. Cartwright, *The Twenty-Four Hour Mind*, 165; M. P. Walker, "Sleep, Memory and Emotion," *Progress in Brain Research* 185 (2010): 49-68, http://www.ncbi.nlm.nih.gov/pubmed/21075233.
8. Cartwright, *The Twenty-Four Hour Mind*, 27.
9. Patricia Cox Miller, *Dreams in Late Antiquity: Studies in the Imagination of a Culture* (Princeton: Princeton University Press, 1994), 86.
10. Robert Stickgold et al. "Sleep-Induced Changes in Associative Memory," *Journal of Cognitive Neuroscience* 11, no. 2 (Mar 1999): 182–93, http://www.mitpressjournals.org/doi/abs/10.1162/089892999563319.
11. Division of Sleep Medicine, "To Understand the Big Picture, Give it Time—And Sleep," Harvard Medical School Press Release (April 22, 2007), https://sleep.med.harvard.edu/news/120/To+Understand+The+Big+Picture+Give+It+Time+And+Sleep.
12. Deidre Barrett, *The Committee of Sleep*, 89–90.
13. C. M. Den Blanken and E. J. G. Meijer, "An Historical View of Dreams and the Way to Direct Them; Practical Observations by Marie-Jean-Leon Lecoq, Le Marquis d'Hervey-Saint-Denis1," Spiritwatch, accessed April 15, 2013, http://www.sawka.com/spiritwatch/anhis.htm.
14. John Gould, *Myth, Ritual, Memory, and Exchange: Essays in Greek Literature and Culture* (Oxford: Oxford University Press, 2001); Ginette Paris, *Pagan Grace: Dionysus, Hermes and Goddess Memory* (New York: Spring, 1998).

Chapter 11—Knitting Up the "Raveled Sleave of Care": Emotional Restoration

1. Aristotle, *On Dreams*, J.I. Bear, trans. (350 BC), accessed April 18, 2013, http://classics.mit.edu/Aristotle/dreams.html.
2. Owen Flanagan, "Deconstructing Dreams: The Spandrels of Sleep," *The Journal of Philosophy* 92, no. 1 (January 1995): 5–27, http://www.jstor.org/discover/10.2307/2940806?uid=3739816&uid=2&uid=4&uid=3739256&sid=21102045245261; J. Allan Hobson and Robert W. McCarley, "The Brain as a Dream State Generator: An Activation-Synthesis Hypothesis of the Dream Process," *American Journal of Psychiatry* 134, no. 12 (December 1977): 1335–48, http://www.psychology.uiowa.edu/faculty/blumberg/Course_Docs/Seminar.2008/Readings/Hobson.McCarley.pdf.
3. Rosalind Cartwright et al., "Relation of Dreams to Waking Concerns," *Psychiatry Research* 141, no. 3 (March 30, 2006): 261-70, http://www.ncbi.nlm.nih.gov/pubmed/16497389, Mark Balgrave, "Dreams as the Reflection of Our Waking Concerns and Abilities: A Critique of the Problem-Solving Paradigm in Dream Research," *Dreaming: Journal of the Association for the Study of Dreams* 2, no. 4 (December, 1992): 205–20, http://www.asdreams.org/journal/issues/asdj2-04.htm.
4. Cartwright, *The Twenty-Four Hour Mind*, 165; Nicholas D. J. Peterson et al., "Limbic System Function and Dream Content in University Students," *The Journal of Neuropsychiatry and the Neurosciences* 14, no. 3 (August 1, 2002), http://neuro.psychiatryonline.org/article.aspx?articleID=101716; "What Are Dreams? Psychologists and Brain Scientists Have New Answers to an Age-Old Question," *NOVA* (June 29, 2011), http://www.pbs.org/wgbh/nova/body/what-are-dreams.html.
5. Cartwright, *The Twenty-Four Hour Mind*, 55–71.
6. Mathew P. Walker, "Overnight Therapy? The Role of Sleep in Emotional Brain Processing," *Psychological Bulletin* 135, no. 5 (2009): 731–48, http://walkerlab.berkeley.edu/reprints/WalkerVanDerHelm_PsychBull_2009.pdf.
7. Patricia Cox Miller, *Dreams in Late Antiquity: Studies in the Imagination of a Culture* (Princeton: Princeton University Press, 1994), 128.
8. Els van der Helm, Ninad Gujar, and Matthew P. Walker, "Sleep Deprivation Impairs the Accurate Recognition of Human Emotions," *Sleep* 33, no. 3 (March 1, 2010): 335–42, http://www.ncbi.nlm.nih.gov/pmc/articles/PMC2831427/.

9. Seung-Schik Yoo et al., "The Human Emotional Brain Without Sleep—A Prefrontal Amygdala Disconnect," *Current Biology* 17, no. 20 (2007): R877–R878, http://www.cell.com/current-biology/abstract/S0960-9822%2807%2901783-6.
10. Dag Neckelmann, Amstein Mykletun, and Alv A. Dahl, "Chronic Insomnia as a Risk Factor for Developing Anxiety and Depression," *Sleep* 30, no. 7 (July 1, 2007): 873–80, http://www.ncbi.nlm.nih.gov/pmc/articles/PMC1978360/.
11. T. R. Goldstein, J. A. Bridge, and D. A. Brent, "Sleep Disturbance Preceding Completed Suicide in Adolescents," *Journal of Consulting and Clinical Psychology* 76, no. 1 (February 2008), http://www.ncbi.nlm.nih.gov/pubmed/18229986; Rebecca A. Bernert and Thomas E. Joiner, "Sleep Disturbances and Suicide Risk: A Review of the Literature," *Neuropsychiatric Disease and Treatment* 3, no. 6 (December 2007), 735–43, http://www.ncbi.nlm.nih.gov/pmc/articles/PMC2656315/.
12. "Tired and Edgy? Sleep Deprivation Boosts Anticipatory Anxiety," *Science Daily*, June 26, 2013, http://www.sciencedaily.com/releases/2013/06/130626143031.htm.
13. Pearl Marshall and Margaret Studer, "Enthroned at 4, Exiled at 23, Tibet's Dalai Lama Visits the U.S., but Can He Go Home Again?," *People* (September 10, 1979), www.people.com/people/article/0,,20074531,oo.html.
14. Meir H. Kryger, "PTSD and Sleep," National Sleep Foundation, March 8, 2013, http://www.sleepfoundation.org/article/ptsd-and-sleep.
15. Madeleine Kruhly, "No Rest for the Haunted: Sleep May Actually Reinforce Bad Memories," *Atlantic*, June 27, 2012, http://www.theatlantic.com/health/archive/2012/06/no-rest-for-the-haunted-sleep-may-actually-reinforce-bad-memories/259053/.
16. Shlomi Cohen et al., "Post-Exposure Sleep Deprivation Facilitates Correctly Timed Interactions Between Glucocorticoid and Adrenergic Systems, Which Attenuate Traumatic Stress Responses," *Neuropsychopharmacology* 37 (2012): 2388-2404, http://www.nature.com/npp/journal/v37/n11/full/npp201294a.html.
17. David Levine, "Why Sleep Deprivation Eases Depression," *Scientific American*, April 26, 2013, http://www.scientificamerican.com/article.cfm?id=why-sleep-deprivation-eases-depression.
18. Susan Donaldson James, "Scientists Probe Sleep Deprivation, Depression Links," CBS News, August 31, 2013, http://abcnews.go.com/Health/Sleep/sleep-deprivation-helps-depressed-scientists/story?id=11516912#.

UdCsG_k4t-c.

19. M. Ansseau, "Benzodiazepines and Sleep," *Acta Psychiatrica Belgica* 85, no. 4 (July–August 1985): 522–32, http://www.ncbi.nlm.nih.gov/pubmed/2865871.
20. Bettye Miller, "Sleep Mechanism Identified That Plays Role in Emotional Memory," *UCR Today*, June 12, 2013, http://ucrtoday.ucr.edu/15887.
21. Hara Estroff Marano, "Bedfellows: Insomnia and Depression," *Psychology Today*, July 1, 2003, http://www.psychologytoday.com/articles/200307/bedfellows-insomnia-and-depression; D. J. Taylor et al., "Epidemiology of Insomnia, Depression, and Anxiety," *Sleep* 28, no. 11 (November 2005): 1457–64, http://www.ncbi.nlm.nih.gov/pubmed/16335332; Matthew Edlund, "The Power of Rest," *Psychology Today*, April 7, 2011, http://www.psychologytoday.com/blog/the-power-rest/201104/is-depression-making-me-sleepless-or-is-insomnia-making-me-depressed-0.
22. Gregory Stores, "Misdiagnosing Sleep Disorders as Primary Psychiatric Conditions," *Advances in Psychiatric Treatment* 9 (2003): 69–77, http://apt.rcpsych.org/content/9/1/69.short.
23. Rosalind D. Cartwright, "Sleepwalking and State of Mind in the Courtroom," in *The Twenty-Four Hour Mind*, 113–26.
24. David M. Eagleman, "The Brain on Trial," *Atlantic*, July–August 2011, http://www.theatlantic.com/magazine/archive/2011/07/the-brain-on-trial/308520/.
25. Phillippe Goddin, *The Art of Hergé, Inventor of Tintin: Volume 1: 1907–1937*, trans. Michael Farr (San Francisco: Last Gasp, 2008), 656-57.
26. Deirdre Barrett and Patrick McNamara, *The Encyclopedia of Sleep and Dreams: The Evolution, Function, Nature and Mysteries of Slumber* (Santa Barbara, CA: ABC-CLIO, 2012), 403.
27. Anne Mancini, *The Intelligence of Dreams* (Buenos Aires: Buenos Books America, 2004), 154.
28. Sarvananda Bluestone, *The World Dream Book: Use the Wisdom of World Cultures to Uncover Your Dream Power* (Rochester, VT: Inner Traditions, 2002), 107.
29. Melinda Beck, "How to Tame Your Nightmares," *Wall Street Journal*, July 20, 2010, http://online.wsj.com/article/SB10001424052748703720504575376994152084232.html.
30. Ernest Hartmann, "The Nightmare Is the Most Useful Dream," Ernest Hartmann: Selected Papers to 2013, accessed August 15, 2013, http://ernesthartmann.org/ERNEST_HARTMANN_MD/HOME.html.
31. Kelly Bulkeley, "Lyndon B. Johnson's Dreams," *Dream Research &*

Education (blog), October 2, 2009, http://kellybulkeley.org/lyndon-johnson-dreams/.

Chapter 12—Sleep Has No Master: Subversive Dreaming

1. Li, "Playing with the Clouds."
2. Roger Ivar Lohmann, "Supernatural Encounters of the Asabano in Two Traditions and Three States of Consciousness," in *Dream Travelers: Sleep Experiences and Culture in the Western Pacific*, ed. Roger Ivar Lohmann (New York: Palgrave MacMillan, 2003), 189.
3. Ibn Khaldun, *The Muqaddimah: An Introduction to History*, trans. Franz Rosenthal (Princeton: Princeton University Press, 1969), 81.
4. Waud Kracke, "Beyond the Mythologies: A Shape of Dreaming," in *Dream Travelers*, ed. Lohman, 2011.
5. William Dement and Nathanial Kleitman, "The Relation of Eye Movements During Sleep to Dream Activity: An Objective Method for the Study of Dreaming," *Journal of Experimental Psychology* 53, no. 5 (May, 1957), http://www.ncbi.nlm.nih.gov/pubmed/1342894.
6. Amish S. Dave and Daniel Margoliash, "Song Replay During Sleep and Computational Rules for Sensorimotor Vocal Learning," *Science* 290, no. 5492 (October 27, 2000): 812–16, http://www.ncbi.nlm.nih.gov/pubmed/11052946.
7. "Koko's Mourning for Michael," Koko's World, August 2, 2000, http://www.koko.org/world/mourning_koko.html.
8. Juliette Harrisson, "The Classical Greek Practice of Incubation and Some Near Eastern Predecessors," Academia, accessed April 15, 2013, http://www.academia.edu/277934/The_Classical_Greek_Practice_of_Incubation_and_some_Near_Eastern _Predecessors.
9. "Two Dreams and a Sleepless Night: A Night in a Mayan Dream House," Living in the Mayan Cholq'ij, http://www.witzmountain.com/2012_Dreamhouse.html.
10. Lee Ann Obringer, "How Dreams Work," How Stuff Works, http://science.howstuffworks.com/life/inside-the-mind/human-brain/dream4.htm.
11. Ulu Temay, quoted in S. Valadez, "Dreams and Visions from the Gods: An Interview with Ulu Temay, Huichol Shaman," *Shaman's Drum* 6 (1986): 18–23.
12. Sarah Bradford, *Harriet Tubman: The Moses of Her People* (Bedford, MA: Applewood, 1993), 114.

13. Beverly Lowry, *Her Dream of Dreams: The Rise and Triumph of Madam C. J. Walker* (New York: Random House, 2003).
14. Leyma Gbowee, "Gbowee Talks About Winning Nobel Peace Prize," National Public Radio, October 7, 2011, http://www.npr.org/2011/10/07/141162208/gbowee-talks-about-winning-nobel-peace-prize.
15. Robert L. Van de Castle, *Our Dreaming Mind* (New York: Random House, 1994), 30.
16. "Dream," Merriam Webster Dictionary, accessed April 17, 2013, http://www.merriamwebster.com/dictionary/dream.
17. Robert L. Van de Castle, *Our Dreaming Mind* (New York: Random House, 1994), 30.
18. Ralph L. Woods, Herbert B. Greenhouse, eds., *The New World of Dreams*, (New York: MacMillan, 1974), 135–6.
19. Kelly Bulkeley, *Spiritual Dreaming: A Cross-Cultural and Historical Journey* (New York: Paulist Press, 1995), 175–6.
20. Edgar Cayce, *Dreams & Visions* (Virginia Beach: A.R.E., 2009), 19.
21. Thomas Mann, *The Magic Mountain* (London: Vintage, 1996), 495.
22. D. Kahn, S. Krippner, and A. Combs, "Dreaming and the Self-Organizing Brain," *Journal of Consciousness Studies* 7, no. 7 (2000): 4–11, http://www.ingentaconnect.com/content/imp/jcs/2000/00000007/00000007/1112?crawler=true; Stanley Krippner, Ruth Richards, and Frederick David Abraham, "Creativity and Chaos in Waking and Dreaming States," *NeuroQuantology* 10, no. 2 (2012): 164–76, http://www.neuroquantology.com/index.php/journal/article/view/563#.UXB3kbU4uHg.
23. Jorges Luis Borges, "Nightmares," in *Seven Nights*, trans. Eliot Weinberger (Fondo de Cultura Económica, 1980), 26–41.
24. Kelly Bulkeley, *Spiritual Dreaming: A Cross-Cultural and Historical Journey* (Mahwah, NJ: Paulist, 1995), 36.
25. Carl Jung, "The Meaning of Psychology for Modern Man," in *Collected Works of C. G. Jung*, vol. 10, *Civilization in Transition*, trans. Gerhard Adler (Princeton: Princeton University Press, 1970), 324.

Chapter 13—Ordinary Dreams: When One Hand Washes the Other

1. William Golding, *Pincher Martin: The Two Deaths of Christopher Martin* (New York: Mariner Books, 2002), chapter 6.
2. Nathaniel Bland, "Muhammedan Tabir, or Dream Interpretation," in

Ralph L. Woods, Herbert Greenhouse, eds., *The New World of Dreams* (New York: MacMillan, 1974), 131–5.

3. Naomi Epel, *Writers Dreaming* (New York: Carol Southern, 1993), 139.
4. C.G. Jung, *Two Essays on Analytical Psychology: Collected Works of C.G. Jung* Vol. 7 (Princeton: Princeton University Press, 1977) 100–101.
5. Cartwright, *The Twenty-Four Hour Mind*, 165.
6. Norbu Namkhai Norbu, *Dream Yoga and the Practice of Natural Light*, ed. Michael Katz (Boston: Snow Lion, 1992), 37–42.
7. Epel, *Writers Dreaming*, 13.
8. Oliver Sacks, *Awakenings* (New York: Dutton, 1983), 67–79.
9. C.G. Jung, *The Archetypal and the Collective Unconscious: Collected Works of C.G. Jung*, Vol. 9, Part 1 (Princeton: Princeton University Press, 1981).
10. Thomas Mann, *The Magic Mountain*, 495.
11. Marina Roseman, *Healing Sounds from the Malaysian Rainforest: Temiar Music and Medicine* (Berkeley: University of California Press, 1993), 177; Rane Willerslev, *Soul Hunter: Hunting, Animism, and Personhood Among the Siberian Yukaghirs* (Berkeley: University of California Press, 2007), 175–76; Roger Ivar Lohmann, *Dream Travelers: Sleep Experiences and Culture in the Western Pacific* (England: Palgrave Macmillan, 2003), 15.
12. Vincent Crapanzano, *Hermes' Dilemma and Hamlet's Desire: On the Epistemology of Interpretation* (Cambridge, MA: Harvard University Press, 1992), 142.
13. Amira Mittermaier, *Dreams That Matter: Egyptian Landscapes of the Imagination* (Berkeley: University of California Press, 2011), 15.
14. G. Berlucchi and H. A. Buchtel, "Neuronal Plasticity: Historical Roots and Evolution of Meaning, *Experimental Brain Research* 192, no. 3 (January, 2009): 307–19.
15. Susana Valadez, "An Interview with Ulu Temay, Huichol Shaman," *Shaman's Drum 6* (1986), 19, quoted in Marc Ian Barasch, *Healing Dreams: Exploring the Dreams That Can Transform Your Life* (New York: Penguin, 2000), 36.
16. Harmon Bro, *Edgar Cayce on Dreams* (Modesto, CA: Castle Books, 1968), excerpted at: http://www.terrygillisdreamanalyst.ca/Cayce.pdf.
17. Reb Yakov Leib HaKohain, "Kaballah and the Interpretation of Dreams," in *Modern Jew in Search of a Soul*, ed. J. Marvin Spiegelman (Las Vegas: Falcon, 1986), http://www.donmeh-west.com/intrpdrms.shtml.
18. Florence Brunois, "Man or Animal: Who Copies Who? Interspecific

Empathy and Imitation Among the Kasua of New Guinea," in *Animal Names*, Alessandro Minelli, Gherardo Ortalli, Glauco Sanga, eds. (Venice: Instituto Veneto di Scienze Lettere ed Arti, 2004).

19. S. F. R. Price, "The Future of Dreams: From Freud to Artemidorus," *Past & Present* 113 (Nov. 1986): 3–37.
20. James Hillman, *The Dream and the Underworld* (New York: Harper and Row, 1979), 96–7.
21. Lohmann, *Dream Travelers*, 15.
22. Ellen Basso, "The Implications of a Progressive Theory of Dreaming," in *Dreaming*, ed. Barbara Tedlock, 92–5.
23. Tina Hesman Saey, "The Why of Sleep," *Science News*, October 24, 2009, 17, http://www.sciencenews.org/pictures/sleep/sn_sleep_fulledition_lo.pdf.
24. Harry T. Hunt, *The Multiplicity of Dreams: Memory, Imagination, and Consciousness* (New Haven, CT: Yale University Press, 1991), 133.
25. Chogyal Namkhai Norbu, *Dream Yoga and the Practice of Natural Light*, Michael Katz, ed. (Ithica, NY: Snow Lion, 2002).
26. Dean Radin, *Entangled Minds: Extrasensory Experiences in a Quantum Reality* (New York: Simon and Schuster, 2006), 21.
27. William C. Chittick, "Meeting with Imaginal Men," *Sufi* 19, accessed September 7, 2013, http://www.sufism.ru/eng/txts/a_meetings.htm.
28. Jay Bregman, *Synesius of Cyrene: Philosopher-Bishop* (Berkeley: University of California Press, 1982), 148.

Chapter 14—Big Dreams: Encounters with the Other Side

1. Tedlock, *Dreaming*; Lohman, *Dream Travelers*.
2. William Dement, *Some Must Watch While Some Must Sleep* (San Francisco: W. H. Freeman, 1972), 102.
3. Mittermaier, *Dreams That Matter*.
4. Epel, *Writers Dreaming*, 209–18.
5. Mittermaier, *Dreams That Matter*, 139.
6. Lady Sarashina, *As I Crossed a Bridge of Dreams: Recollections of a Woman in Eleventh-Century Japan*, Ivan Morris, trans. (New York: Penguin, 1975).
7. Edward Hoffman, *Visions of Innocence* (Boston: Shambhala, 1992), 162–3.
8. Bulkeley, *Spiritual Dreaming*, 36.
9. Simo Knuttila, "Medieval Theories of Future Contingents," *Stanford*

Encyclopedia of Philosophy, 2011, http://plato.stanford.edu/entries/medieval-futcont/.

10. C.G. Jung, "General Aspects of Dream Psychology," *The Structure and Dynamics of the Psyche: Collected Works of C. G. Jung*, Vol. 8 (Princeton: Princeton University Press, 1960), 493.
11. Rosalind Cartwright and Lynn Lamberg, *Crisis Dreaming: Using Your Dreams to Solve Your Problems* (New York: Harper Collins, 1992), 269.
12. "President Dreams of Crash," *The Age*, June 3, 1938, http://news.google.com/newspapers?nid=1300&dat=19380603&id=Ap1VAAAAIBAJ&sjid=J5cDAAAAIBAJ&pg=3511,3893714.
13. Li, "Dreams of Interpretation," 37.
14. Theodora Kroeber and Robert F. Heizer, *Almost Ancestors: The First Californians* (San Francisco: Sierra Club, 1968).

Chapter 15—Waking Up Is Hard to Do: Internal and Social Time

1. William J. H. Andrewes, "A Brief History of Clocks," *Scientific American*, January 15, 2012, http://www.scientificamerican.com/article.cfm?id=a-chronicle-of-timekeeping; "History of Clocks," History World, http://www.historyworld.net/wrldhis/plaintexthistories.asp?historyid=ac08.
2. Michael Menaker, "Special Topic: Circadian Rhythms," *Annual Review of Physiology* 55 (1993): 657-9, http://millar.bio.ed.ac.uk/andrewM/CBT%20tutorial/HISTBACK.html.
3. Till Roenneberg, *Internal Time*, 78–80.
4. Ibid., 114–28.
5. Ibid., 129–38.
6. Melissa Lee Phillips, "Circadian Rhythms: Of Owls, Larks and Alarm Clocks," *Nature* 458 (March 11, 2009): 142–4, http://www.nature.com/news/2009/090311/full/458142a.html.
7. "Dawn Chorus," *Royal Society for the Protection of Birds*, accessed September 5, 2013, http://www.arranbirding.co.uk/dawn_chorus.html.
8. Ryan Jaslow, "'Social Jet Lag' Is a Problem for Most of Us, and It's Fueling the Obesity Epidemic, Study Suggests," CBS News, May 11, 2012, http://www.cbsnews.com/8301-504763_162-57432660-10391704/social-jet-lag-is-a-problem-for-most-of-us-and-its-fueling-the-obesity-epidemic-study-suggests/.
9. Sloan Work and Family Research Network, "Questions and Answers about Shift Work: A Sloan Work and Family Research Network Fact

Sheet," last updated September 2009, https://workfamily.sas.upenn.edu/sites/workfamily.sas.upenn.edu/files/imported/pdfs/shiftwork.pdf.

10. T. Roth, "Shift Work Disorder: Overview and Diagnosis," *Journal of Clinical Psychiatry* 73, no. 3 (March 2012): e09, http://www.ncbi.nlm.nih.gov/pubmed/22490262.
11. Chris Hanlon, "Snoozing at Your Desk? Piling on the Pounds? You May Have Social Jet Lag," *Daily Mail*, May 10, 2012, http://www.dailymail.co.uk/health/article-2142522/Are-suffering-social-jetlag-Rising-levels-sleep-deprivation-blamed-mismatch-body-clock-reality-daily-lives.html.
12. Lin Fritschi, "Shift Work and Cancer," *Medscape Today*, 2009, http://www.medscape.com/viewarticle/707460.
13. American Academy of Sleep Medicine, "Circadian Rhythm Sleep Disorders," accessed April 24, 2013, http://www.aasmnet.org/resources/factsheets/crsd.pdf.
14. H. R. Colten and B. M. Altevogt, eds., "Functional and Economic Impact of Sleep Loss and Sleep-Related Disorders," in *Sleep Disorders and Sleep Deprivation: An Unmet Public Health Problem* (Washington, DC: National Academies Press, 2006), http://www.ncbi.nlm.nih.gov/books/NBK19958/.
15. Sarah Spinks, "Adolescents and Sleep," *Frontline*, PBS, accessed April 24, 2013, http://www.pbs.org/wgbh/pages/frontline/shows/teenbrain/from/sleep.html.
16. Siri Carpenter, "Sleep Deprivation May Be Undermining Teen Health," *American Psychological Association Monitor* 32, no. 9 (October 2001): 42.
17. Bryan D. Palmer, *Cultures of Darkness: Night Travels in the Histories of Transgression* (New York: Monthly Review Press, 2000).
18. Josemaría Escrivá, "Mortification," *The Way* (London: Scepter Publications, 1992), 191, www.escrivaworks.org/book/the_way-chapter-6.htm.
19. Robertson Davies, *The Papers of Samuel Marchbanks* (London: Viking, 1986), 76.
20. Miranda Hitti, "Morning Grogginess Worse Than No Sleep," WebMD Health News, January 10, 2006, http://www.webmd.com/sleep-disorders/news/20060110/morning-grogginess-worse-than-no-sleep.
21. C. Marzano et al., "Electroencephalographic Sleep Inertia of the Awakening Brain," *Neuroscience* 176 (March 10, 2011): 308–17, http://www.ncbi.nlm.nih.gov/pubmed/21167917; Gilberte Hofer-Tinguely et al., "Sleep Inertia: Performance Changes After Sleep, Rest and Active Waking," *Cognitive Brain Research* 22, no. 3 (March, 2005): 323–31,

http://www.sciencedirect.com/science/article/pii/S0926641004002708.

22. Brandon Peters, "How Does Sleep Inertia Make It Hard to Wake Up?" About.com, updated March 1, 2013, http://sleepdisorders.about.com/od/doihaveasleepdisorder/f/Sleep_Inertia.htm.
23. Hofer-Tinguely et al., "Sleep Inertia."
24. Hitti, "Morning Grogginess Worse Than No Sleep."
25. Brian Palmer, "Not Guilty by Reason of Grogginess," *Slate*, February 20, 2013, http://www.slate.com/articles/health_and_science/explainer/2013/02/oscar_pistorius_could_sleepiness_have_caused_him_to_mistake_reeva_steenkamp.html.
26. J. E. Cosnett, "Charles Dickens: Observer of Sleep and Its Disorders," Sleep 15, no. 3 (June 1992): 264–7, http://www.ncbi.nlm.nih.gov/pubmed/1621029.
27. Stephen LaBerge and Howard Rheingold, *Exploring the World of Lucid Dreaming* (New York: Ballantine, 1997); Robert Waggoner, *Lucid Dreaming: Gateway to the Inner Self* (Needham, MA: Moment Point, 2008); Tenzin Wangyol Rimpoche, *The Tibetan Yogas of Dream and Sleep* (Boston: Snow Lion, 1998); Barbara Tedlock, "Sharing and Interpreting Dreams in Amerindian Nations," *Dream Cultures*, eds. David Shulman and Guy G. Stroumsa, 87–103.
28. Jeff Warren, *The Head Trip: Adventures on the Wheel of Consciousness* (New York: Random House, 2007), 22.
29. Rumi, *Unseen Rain*, trans. Coleman Barks, The Threshold Society, accessed April 24, 2013, http://sufism.org/lineage/rumi/rumi-excerpts/poems-of-rumi-tr-by-coleman-barks-published-by-threshold-books-2.
30. T. Akerstedt et al., "The Meaning of Good Sleep: A Longitudinal Study of Polysomnography and Subjective Sleep Quality," *Journal of Sleep Research* 3, no. 3 (September, 1994): 152–8, http://www.ncbi.nlm.nih.gov/pubmed/10607120; "The Perfect Sleep," *National Post* (June 24, 2006), http://www.canada.com/nationalpost/story.html?id=bff37852-a5d6-4bd7-918c-a74b409e5339.
31. Ann Faraday, quoted in John Aske, "Dreams: The Forest of the Night," *Buddhism Now* (January 1, 2013), http://buddhismnow.com/2013/01/01/dreams-by-john-aske/.
32. Sri Aurobindo and the Mother, selections compiled by A.S. Dalal, *The Yoga of Sleep and Dreams: The Night-School of Sadhana* (Twin Lakes, WI: Lotus, 2004), 1–22, 38–56.
33. Richard King, *Early Advaita Vedanta and Buddhism: The Mahayana Context of Guadapadiya-Karika* (Albany: State University of New York

Press, 1995); Pravrajika Brahmaprana, "Consciousness in Advaita Vedanta," Hindupedia (last updated May 19, 2010), http://www.hindupedia.com/en/Consciousness_in_Advaita_Vedanta.

Chapter 16—Enamored with Wakefulness: Phasing Out Sleep

1. Grace Wing Slick, "White Rabbit," Jefferson Airplane, University Music Publishing Group, 1967.
2. "FDA Approves of Expanded Labelling of Provigil (Modafinil), Previously Approved for Treatment of Narcolepsy," DocGuide, January 26, 2004, http://www.docguide.com/fda-approves-expanded-labelling-provigil-modafinil-previously-approved-treatment-narcolepsy.
3. Dan Harris, Lana Zak, and Mark Abdelmalek, "Provigil: The Secret to Success?" ABC News, July 17, 2012, http://abcnews.go.com/Health/provigil-secret-success/story?id=16788001#.UXSSF7U4uHg; Julia Layton, "Is Science Phasing Out Sleep?" How Stuff Works, accessed April 21, 2013, http://science.howstuffworks.com/life/sleep-is-so-last-year.htm.
4. Pendergrast, *Uncommon Grounds*, 12.
5. "Caffeine: Consumption by Country," EnergyFiend, accessed April 21, 2013, http://www.energyfiend.com/caffeine-what-the-world-drinks.
6. David Plotz, "Wake Up, Little Susie," *Slate*, March 7, 2003, http://www.slate.com/articles/health_and_science/superman/2003/03/wake_up_little_susie.3.html.
7. Maia Szalavitz, "Popping Smart Pills: The Case for Cognitive Enhancement," *Time*, January 6, 2009, http://www.time.com/time/health/article/0,8599,1869435,00.html.
8. Barbara Sahakian and Sharon Morein-Zamir, "Professor's Little Helper," *Nature* 450 (December 20, 2007): 1157–9, http://www.nature.com/nature/journal/v450/n7173/full/4501157a.html.
9. Akito Hisanaga et al., "A Case of Sub Wakefulness Syndrome," *Psychiatry and Clinical Neurosciences* 52, no. 2 (April 1998): 206–7, http://onlinelibrary.wiley.com/doi/10.1111/j.1440-1819.1998.tb01033.x/abstract; "Definition of Excessive Daytime Sleepiness," MedicineNet, last updated June 14, 2012), http://www.medterms.com/script/main/art.asp?articlekey=10472.
10. "Stress May Lead Students to Use Stimulants," *Science Daily*, April 11, 2008, http://www.sciencedaily.com/releases/2008/04/080407195349.

htm.

11. Alexis Madrigal, "Wired.com Readers' Brain-Enhancing Drug Regimens," *Wired*, April 24, 2008, http://www.wired.com/medtech/drugs/news/2008/04/smart_drugs?currentPage=all.
12. Brad Knickerbocker, "Military Looks to Drugs for Battle Readiness," *Christian Science Monitor*, August 9, 2002, http://www.csmonitor.com/2002/0809/p01s04-usmi.html; Susan Donaldson James, "Super Soldiers? Military Drug Is Rage Among Students, Young Professionals," ABC News, July 24, 2007, http://abcnews.go.com/Technology/Health/story?id=3408266&page=1#.UXTNybU4uHh.
13. Richard Martin, "It's Wake-up Time," *Wired*, November 2003, http://www.wired.com/wired/archive/11.11/sleep.html.
14. Graham Lawton, "Get Ready for 24-Hour Living," *New Scientist*, February 18, 2006, http://www.newscientist.com/article/mg18925391.300.
15. Alexis Madrigal, "Snorting a Brain Chemical Could Replace Sleep," *Wired*, December 28, 2007, http://www.wired.com/science/discoveries/news/2007/12/sleep_deprivation.
16. Ullrich Wagner et al., "Sleep Inspires Insight," *Nature* 427 (January 22, 2004): 352–5, http://www.nature.com/nature/journal/v427/n6972/abs/nature02223.html.
17. Evelyn Pringle, "The Rise and Fall of Provigil—Part I," *Salient News*, September 20, 2010, http://www.salient-news.com/2010/09/provigil-cephalo/.
18. Amy Barrett, "This Pep Pill Is Pushing Its Luck," *Bloomberg Businessweek Magazine*, October 31, 2004, http://www.businessweek.com/stories/2004-10-31/this-pep-pill-is-pushing-its-luck.
19. Michael Carrier, "Provigil: A Case Study of Anticompetitive Behavior," *Hastings Science and Technology Law Journal* 441 (August 31, 2011), http://hstlj.org/articles/provigil-a-case-study-of-anticompetitive-behavior/.

Chapter 17—Waking Up Again: Doubt, Certainty, and the Future of Sleep

1. Sharma, *Sleep as a State of Consciousness in Advaita Vedanta*, 44.
2. Richard King, *Early Advaita Vedanta and Buddhism: The Mahayana Context of Guadapadiya-Karika* (Albany, NY: State University of New York Press, 1995); Walpola Rahula, "Alayavijnana—Store Consciousness," *Buddhism Today*, accessed April 26, 2013, http://www.buddhismtoday.

com/english/philosophy/maha/032-Alayavijnana.htm.

3. C.G. Jung, "The Practical Use of Dream Analysis," *The Practice of Psychotherapy: Collected Works of C. G. Jung*, Vol. 16 (Princeton: Princeton University Press, 1981), 125.
4. Rodolfo R. Llinás and Urs Ribary, "Perception as an Oneiric-Like State Modulated by the Senses," in *Large-Scale Neuronal Theories of the Brain*, eds. Christof Koch and Joel L. Davis (Boston: MIT Press, 1994), 111.
5. V. S. Ramachandran and Sandra Blakeslee, *Phantoms in the Brain: Probing the Mysteries of the Human Mind* (New York: HarperCollins, 1999), 112.
6. Terry Eagleton, *The Meaning of Life: A Very Short Introduction* (Oxford: Oxford University Press, 2007), 62.
7. Bill Clinton (speech, University of California, Berkeley, CA, January 29, 2002), http://www.berkeley.edu/news/features/2002/clinton/clinton-transcript.html.
8. Amanda Gardner, "Is a Better Sleeping Pill on the Way?" WebMD, April 3, 2013, http://www.webmd.com/sleep-disorders/news/20130403/is-a-better-sleeping-pill-on-the-way.
9. Toni Clarke, "Suvorexant, Insomnia Drug, Moves Step Closer to Approval by FDA," *Huffington Post*, May 22, 2013, http://www.huffingtonpost.com/2013/05/23/suvorexant-sleeping-pill-insomnia-drug-fda_n_3322733.html.
10. Sam A. Deadwiler et al., "Systematic and Nasal Delivery of Orexin-A (Hypocretin-1) Reduces of Effects of Sleep Deprivation on Cognitive Performance in Nonhuman Primates," *The Journal of Neuroscience* 27, no. 52 (December 26, 2007): 14239–47, http://www.jneurosci.org/content/27/52/14239.abstract; Madrigal, "Snorting a Brain Chemical Could Replace Sleep."
11. Madrigal, "Snorting a Brain Chemical Could Replace Sleep."

RECOMMENDED READING

Adler, Shelley R. *Sleep Paralysis: Night-Mares, Nocebos, and the Mind-Body Connection*. New Brunswick, NJ: Rutgers University Press, 2010.

Barrett, Deidre, and Patrick McNamara. *The Encyclopedia of Sleep and Dreams: The Evolution, Function, Nature, and Mysteries of Slumber*. Westport, CT: Greenwood Publishing Group, 2012.

Bulkeley, Kelly. *Dreaming in the World's Religions: A Comparative History*. New York: New York University Press, 2008.

Butler, Blake. *Nothing: A Portrait of Insomnia*. New York: Harper Collins, 2011.

Cartwright, Rosalind D. *The Twenty-Four Hour Mind: The Role of Sleep and Dreaming in Our Emotional Lives*. New York: Oxford University Press, 2010.

Ekirch, A. Roger. *At Day's Close: Night in Times Past*. New York: W. W. Norton, 2005.

Flygare, Julie. *Wide Awake and Dreaming: A Memoir of Narcolepsy*. Arlington, VA: Mill Pond Swan Publishing, 2012.

Greene, Gayle. *Insomniac*. Berkeley: University of California Press, 2008.

Hobson, J. Allan. *Dream Life: An Experimental Memoir*. Boston: MIT Press, 2011.

Hufford, David J. *The Terror That Comes in the Night: An Experience-Centered Study of Supernatural Assault Traditions*. Philadelphia: University of Pennsylvania Press, 1989.

Lacrampe, Corine. *Sleep and Rest in Animals*. Toronto: Firefly, 2003.

Lewis, Penelope. *The Secret World of Sleep: The Surprising Science of the Mind at Rest.* New York: Palgrave MacMillan, 2013.

Liedloff, Jean. *The Continuum Concept: In Search of Happiness.* Cambridge: De Capo Press, 1986.

Mageo, Jeanette Marie, ed. *Dreaming and the Self: New Perspectives on Subjectivity, Identity and Emotion* (SUNY Series in Dream Studies). Albany, NY: State University of New York, 2003.

Messer, Jane, ed. *Bedlam: An Anthology of Sleepless Nights.* St. Leonards, Australia: Allen & Unwin, 1997.

Mollison, James. *Where Children Sleep.* Charlottesville, VA: Chris Boot, 2010.

Moss, Robert. *The Secret History of Dreaming.* Novato, CA: New World Library, 2010.

Naiman, Rubin R. *Healing Night: The Science and Spirit of Sleeping, Dreaming, and Awakening.* Minneapolis: Syren, 2006.

Nancy, Jean-Luc. *The Fall of Sleep.* New York: Fordham University Press, 2009.

Randall, David K. *Dreamland: Adventures in the Strange Science of Sleep.* New York: W.W. Norton, 2013.

Roenneberg, Till. *Internal Time: Chronotypes, Social Jet Lag, and Why You're So Tired.* Cambridge, MA: Harvard University Press, 2012.

Small, Meredith F. *Our Babies, Ourselves: How Biology and Culture Shape the Way We Parent.* New York: Anchor, 1998.

Summers-Bremner, Eluned. *Insomnia: A Cultural History.* London: Reaktion, 2008.

Tedlock, Barbara, ed. *Dreaming: Anthropological and Psychological Interpretations.* Santa Fe: School for Advanced Research, 1992.

Williams, Simon J. *Sleep and Society: Sociological Ventures into the (Un) Known.* London: Routledge, 2005.

Wolf-Meyer, Matthew J. *The Slumbering Masses: Sleep, Medicine, and Modern American Life.* Minneapolis: University of Minnesota Press, 2012.

Young, Serinity. *Dreaming in the Lotus: Buddhist Dream Narrative, Imagery and Practice.* Boston: Wisdom, 1999.